Contents

The A–Z Reference Book of Syndromes and Inherited Disorders

Patricia Gilbert

Visiting Senior Lecturer, Warwick University, UK

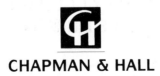

CHAPMAN & HALL

London · Glasgow · Weinheim · New York · Tokyo · Melbourne · Madras

Published by Chapman & Hall, 2–6 Boundary Row, London SE1 8HN, UK

Chapman & Hall, 2–6 Boundary Row, London SE1 8HN, UK

Blackie Academic & Professional, Wester Cleddens Road, Bishopbriggs, Glasgow G64 2NZ, UK

Chapman & Hall GmbH, Pappelallee 3, 69469 Weinheim, Germany

Chapman & Hall USA, 115 Fifth Avenue, New York NY 10003, USA

Chapman & Hall Japan, ITP-Japan, Kyowa Building, 3F, 2–2–1 Hirakawacho, Chiyoda-ku, Tokyo 102, Japan

Chapman & Hall Australia, 102 Dodds Street, South Melbourne, Victoria 3205, Australia

Chapman & Hall India, R. Seshadri, 32 Second Main Road, CIT East, Madras 600 035, India

First edition 1993

Reprinted 1994

Second edition 1996

© 1996 Patricia Gilbert

Phototypeset in 10/12 pt Times by Intype, London

Printed in Great Britain by *Hartnolls Limited, Bodmin, Cornwall*

ISBN 0 412 64120 8

A catalogue record for this book is available from the British Library

Library of Congress Catalog Card Number: 95-70015

∞ Printed on permanent acid-free text paper, manufactured in accordance with ANSI/NISO Z39.48–1992 and ANSI/NISO Z39.48–1984 (Permanence of Paper).

The A–Z Reference Book of Syndromes
and Inherited Disorders

Foreword

More often than not, my heart sinks when I know I am to see a family with a child who has a 'syndrome'. It sinks because it is highly likely that I will not understand the cause of the syndrome, that there will be no specific treatment, that the outlook (particularly in newly-described syndromes) may be unknown and most importantly, the parents will ask me sensible and pertinent questions that I cannot answer. Only if I have special expertise in the disorder or group of disorders, will I be able to help the child as I would wish. Clearly I cannot have expertise in, or knowledge of, even a fraction of the over 2000 syndromes now described.

My difficulties are, I am sure, shared to a greater or lesser extent by all who may be involved in counselling or caring for those disabled by a 'syndrome'. Many who will be responsible for providing for the child's needs, and to whom the parents may turn, may not even have any background medical knowledge. This book, written simply and concisely and in non-technical language, gives just the sort of information needed. It will be a boon to those working in Child Health in the community, in Social Services and in schools.

To cover more than a small selection of the known 'syndromes' is clearly impracticable and to be always up-to-date with the latest 'discovery' in such a rapidly moving field is impossible. Dr Gilbert, with her extensive experience, has chosen wisely and much of the practical information that she gives will not date. Patients, parents and professionals will have reason to be grateful to her for having compiled this compendium on a difficult and important topic.

Professor Dame June Lloyd

Preface

Twenty extra syndromes have been added to the text, bringing the total described to 90. A number of the syndromes added have been specifically requested by readers of the first edition, to whom I give my thanks. The same criteria for inclusion have been applied as in the original text.

The glossary has been substantially extended to include a greater number of perhaps more common medical terms. It is hoped that this will prove helpful to the wider readership.

Where necessary, in the light of further knowledge, additions have been made to the text. Changes have also been made where the addresses of the self-help groups have altered. It is inevitable that this will repeatedly occur over the years. In cases of difficulty, readers should refer to **Contact-a-Family** at 170 Tottenham Court Road, London, W1P 0HA (Tel. 0171 383 3555), who will be able to supply up-to-date information about addresses.

Preface to the first edition

Syndromes are part of everyday diagnosis today. The number described seems to increase weekly. Until now, few were known or documented accurately. Just what are these conditions so labelled?

The Oxford English Dictionary defines a 'syndrome' as 'a concurrence of several symptoms in a disease; a set of such concurrent symptoms'. Put in simpler terms, a 'syndrome' can be described as a specific collection of signs and symptoms which when put together form a recognizable pattern which can be seen to be repeated in another individual.

There are now over 2000 of these syndromes recorded. Some are incredibly rare, others uncommon, whilst others are relatively frequently seen in comparison. For example, in the latter group is Down's syndrome – well-known to most people – with a general incidence of one in approximately every 800 births. Examples of the rarer syndromes are Hunter's and Hurler's syndromes. Both of these syndromes are only found in one child in 100 000. Few doctors, nurses, teachers or social workers (unless their work happens to be with disabled children or adults) will have seen more than a handful of such syndromes. Nevertheless, with the ever-increasing number of syndromes being classified, many of these professionals could well be seeing several people with a specific syndrome during their working lives.

At some time during the lives of people who have a definable syndrome, and most commonly in childhood, help in some form, be it medical, nursing, social or educational, will be needed. In the early days parents will need support, advice and counselling in order to come to terms with their child's disability, as well as the more practical aspects of care. Later in the child's life, social workers and educationalists become involved. All these professionals need accurate knowledge of each specific syndrome if they are to be fully effective in their support of families.

In this book, a small number of the known syndromes are described in alphabetical order. Each section gives guidelines on the practical aspects of help that can be given. Any one of the disciplines of medicine, nursing, social work or education may be involved, but in many cases all four disciplines will have a part to play. Many of the syndromes have self-help groups which have been set up over the years, most frequently by parents who themselves have a child with the specific disorder. Contact points for these self-help groups are to be found at the end of each appropriate section. A basic outline of genetics is given in Appendix A. The effects of a disabling condition on the individual, the family and society in general are also discussed separately. Comprehensive cross-indexing is included to help the reader towards the correct syndrome. For instance, all syndromes having short stature as a characteristic are listed together, as are those syndromes in which a squint might be a factor.

It is hoped that this book will prove to be of value to all professionals who are concerned with the care of disabled children. It has been difficult to limit the syndromes described to a manageable number. The main criteria involved in this choice were two-fold. First, that the syndrome will result in long-term and in many cases life-long problems of one kind or another, either mental or physical. Second, that help is available which can alleviate some of the problems and improve the quality of life. The author will be pleased to receive comments and suggestions as to possible further inclusions for future editions.

Finally, my thanks are due to all the many children with a 'syndrome', and their parents, with whom I have had the privilege to work over the years.

Acknowledgements

My thanks are due to a number of people who have given encouragement and help with the writing of this book. In particular, Dr Terry Billington has given unstintingly of her time and expertise in reading the manuscript. Without her medical and physiotherapy skills much would have been lost. Dr Peter Farndon has also found time in his exceedingly busy life to give advice on genetics for Appendix A, and for this I am in his debt. It must be emphasized that any errors in the text are entirely my own.

Much gratitude is also due to Professor Dame June Lloyd for writing the Foreword to the first edition, and I would like to thank her again for her kind words and sentiments.

Rosemary Morris, Senior Editor at Chapman & Hall, has been unstinting in her enthusiasm and encouragement. Without her ready availability and professional expertise, my task would have been more difficult.

Finally, my thanks again to my husband who has continued to guide me successfully through the minefields of word-processing with patience and cheerfulness.

The effects of disability

Our genetic inheritance colours all our life. The medical conditions passed down the family line will affect our daily lives as surely as does our height, the colour of our skin and our potential for low or high ability. When a syndrome or specifically inherited condition is part of our family tree, these effects can be very great indeed. Our family, our friends and the wider society in which we live will also be affected by our genetic inheritance to a greater or lesser degree. These effects will not cease when childhood is outgrown. The whole of our adult life will be altered, for better or worse.

Between 15% and 20% of adults suffer from some chronic condition which has a bearing on some or all of their daily living. Some of these problems are due, of course, to reasons other than inherited disease. Infection and environmental factors all play their part. But it is thought that some 16% of all babies born alive are born with some defect, many of which are small and insignificant. About half of these will have a condition that will give rise to functional problems of one kind or another throughout their lives. So this aspect of life will have an impact on very many people, whether directly in a day-to-day manner, in the work environment or merely by chance encounter.

Obviously the greatest effect of an inherited disease will be felt by each individual with the specific condition. Every baby has the same basic needs of warmth, food, love and a sense of belonging. The first two of these necessities will be met in all but the most unfortunate of babies. (Although problems of adequate nutrition may cause difficulties in some babies, however, as a result of their genetic inheritance, quite apart from economic factors.) It is love and later, a sense of belonging that some severely disabled babies can lack. Mothers who have waited for nine long months for the arrival of a perfect baby can be distraught at the sight of a disabled newcomer. Careful and sensitive handling of the situation will be needed by those caring for the mother and baby. Under these circumstances, the majority of mothers will accept their baby with love, but a few may take time to come to terms with the unexpected problems facing them. Fortunately, relatively few mothers completely reject their disabled child.

Later in the child's life, problems of acceptance can also occur. This is especially true of the child who has an inherited disorder needing much daily – and possibly nightly – care. Parents can become completely exhausted by the unremitting and inevitable demands of their disabled child. Child abuse in any one of a number of guises may occur, and must be remembered as a possibility under these circumstances. Doctors, nurses and social workers and also teachers when schooldays are reached, should all be aware of the strain under which the parents of a disabled child are living. Help, be it practical, financial or by means of respite care should be made available before the burdens become intolerable.

A further basic need of childhood, and indeed throughout life, is the need to be able to continue to learn. Children with disabilities can often miss out on this vital aspect of normal living. To avoid this, the precise diagnosis of the child's condition must be made initially. Following on from this, assessment of the effects on various functions – vision, hearing and mobility to mention just a few – will be needed. Only then can a specific programme of learning, at whatever basic level, be organized. It is important that the exact nature of the disability is diagnosed early. Vital stages of learning can be missed by this oversight. For example, a baby born with a profound hearing loss will rarely, if ever, be able to speak unless the hearing problem is recognized, and appropriate treatment and training given. Similarly, there are 22 children in every 100 000 in the UK who are registered as blind. These children may have a little residual vision, but this will be too little for the learning process to proceed normally. So suitable educational facilities for learning by methods involving touch must be organized. These are but two examples of the ways in which inherited disease, or a syndrome, can affect an individual's capacity for one of the basic needs of life.

Parents should also be carefully advised on what activities are most suitable for the developmental age of their child. Chronological age, in many syndromes which have a degree of learning disability as part of the symptomatology, is no guide to the stage of development the child has reached. For example, a child with Down's syndrome is frequently behind his/her contemporaries in many aspects of mobility. His/her walking will be delayed due to the almost universal hypotonia found in Down's children. So it is inadvisable for parents to buy toys which are designed for children with early onset of this particular skill. Later, as the child with this disability falls further behind his/her peers, toys and activities will need to be geared to his/her mental abilities rather than to his/her physical age.

A further aspect of life with an inherited disabling condition is the possible need for frequent hospital admissions. This can have two major effects on the life of the individual child. He/she will be away for sometimes long periods of time from his/her immediate family and friends. This can loosen the ties of everyday involvement with work and play. For the older child, when school days are a reality, lessons are also missed unless there can be a close liaison with school, home and hospital. During an acute bout of illness, school work obviously cannot be considered. But during convalescence, time can be spent usefully and happily, catching up with class work. This especially applies to children with such conditions such as cystic fibrosis and osteogenesis imperfecta. In these two conditions (and many others) hospitalization can be a recurrent necessity. All efforts to maintain contact with family and friends should be made.

Finally, when considering the effects of disability on a particular child, appreciation of him/her as an individual must never be forgotten. It is all too easy to talk down to a child in a wheelchair who perhaps has an added speech or hearing problem. It is important, especially as the teenage years are reached, that these young people should be involved in decisions as to their future if at all possible. Whether later schooling should be in a special school or in a mainstream school with added resources involves the child as much as – or perhaps more than – the parents. Choices must be worked out with the child's comments and feelings as an important part of the discussion.

Careers, if applicable, must also be a joint decision between child, parent and advisor. Some disabilities will, of course, prevent any of the more active careers being pursued. But many conditions can allow the sufferer to work alongside their peers with no such disability. Extra consideration for particular activities, such as ramps for those people with a mobility problem or extra light for those with poor vision for instance, may be needed. These, and many other possible complications, must be thought through carefully. But the wishes of the young person should be an important part of the final decision.

To summarize how parents and professionals involved in the care of a child with a disability can make life as normal as possible:

- All efforts should be made to learn as much as possible about the condition from which the child is suffering. Knowing what difficulties the child has to overcome will be half-way to helping him/her to cope with his/her disability. For instance, try to see what life is really like with only central, or 'tunnel', vision by blinkering off the range of side vision with an anorak hood. Crossing the road safely becomes twice as difficult and people coming up quietly behind you can be fairly frightening. Again, tie one arm behind you to find out just how difficult it is to perform many everyday activities with only one functioning arm. These, of course, are gross examples, and easily replicated. How much more difficult is it to understand the problems encountered by children with poor cognitive abilities whose surroundings make little sense to them? But this is just what carers should be trying to do, so that the best possible help can be given.

- Find out how the specific condition may progress. What will the child be doing and feeling when, say, five years have passed. Syndromes and other inherited disorders vary greatly in the way they progress. Some may reach a plateau and stay there for many years, whilst others regrettably progress rapidly. Many syndromes have self-help groups, often started by parents who themselves have a child with the particular condition. Here other sufferers from the same, or a similar, condition can correspond or even meet to compare notes on various problems and how best to overcome them. Friendship, as well as much information on practical aspects of daily living and the benefits obtainable can be gained from such sources.

- All parents have ambitions for their children. When their son or daughter has been found to have a specific disabling condition these ambitions will have to be substantially altered. Sometimes, with a severely affected child, the outlook for life itself is limited. With other serious disorders, parents will be forced to accept that only the most minimal of self-help skills will ever be attained. This can be devastatingly difficult for even the most mature and sympathetic parent, but from the child's point of view it is of immense significance that the adjustment is made. Realistic boundaries can then be set. Here again, sympathetic help from others in similar circumstances can be of enormous value.

- Children who need hospitalization can be prepared for these events. Finding out about admission procedures, what clothing to take, what toys are allowed and many other day-to-day events can do much to alleviate the fear of the unknown. If the parents show a positive attitude to the outcome of the perhaps extended and painful procedures, the upsets of admissions to hospital may be minimized. Whilst the child is actually in hospital, regular visits with small gifts, photographs of family and day-to-day updates of home news can do much to negate feelings of isolation.

  Close liaison with medical and nursing staff regarding the type and length of proposed treatments can help parents explain to their child what is likely to happen to them within the next day or two. Parents are welcome in most hospitals nowadays to be with their child when at all possible during treatment. Parents, for example, are able to be with their child immediately before an anaesthetic, and also to be at their child's side when he/she 'comes round'.

- Diets necessary to the well-being of the disabled child can at times be unpalatable and different from the food their friends are eating. These can be made as palatable as possible and explanations given to friends about the necessity for any restrictions.

- Finally, it must be remembered that children who have a syndrome are twice as likely to have some behavioural disorder as their peers. This is in addition to the effects of the disorder itself. If parents are warned of this and counselled as to how best to avoid these problems, the incidence of outbursts will be reduced to a minimum.

These then are some of the effects an inherited disorder can have on the individual child. But what about the parents who, instead of their hoped-for perfect son or daughter, are faced with a baby who, in addition to looking 'different', has the prospect of needing special, continuing care for many years?

The immediate reaction to the birth of an obviously disabled baby is one of shock and disbelief. Both partners will need sensitive and on-going sympathy and counselling if they are both to accept their baby as he/she is. They must be allowed to grieve, for the birth of a disabled child is surely almost as much a bereavement as a still-birth. All the hopes and aspirations for a perfect, healthy baby are dashed in one brief moment. Parents need time and space to come to terms with their loss. All the usual grief reactions will be there – disbelief, anger, guilt, depression and finally acceptance. These stages will, of course, vary from person to person. Some mothers will find it easy to love and care for their baby, whilst others will find this a traumatic ordeal that has to be worked at for some time. The father, too, must not be forgotten. He may be very supportive, but he, too, will need to work through his disappointment. Thankfully the vast majority of parents come to terms with the outcome of the pregnancy and continue, often for many years, to love and care for their disabled child. Later, as the child grows and possibly becomes more and more demanding of the parents' time and energies, the relationship may be put under severe strain. If there are siblings they can also become resentful of all the attention that is being paid to their disabled brother or sister. These situations need much thought and sensitive counselling to resolve.

Perhaps an even greater shock occurs when the baby appears to be perfect at birth and the genetic disorder only begins to show itself in the first few months or years of life. Hunter's syndrome is an example of this, the baby being normal at birth, but physical and mental deterioration arise at around 18 months to two years of age. Diagnosis will serve to confirm fears of an inherited disorder. Parents will then go through similar grief reactions as other parents who have a child with a genetic disorder which is obvious at birth, such as Down's syndrome or Apert's syndrome, for example.

Genetic disorders can also generate a good deal of guilty feelings in the parents. They feel that it is their fault that their child has been born with the particular syndrome. Again, explanation of the ways of genetic inheritance can help to overcome some of these feelings.

The wider family, not to mention close friends (who may also be in the reproductive years themselves) will be affected by the birth, or subsequent development of a disabled child. Parents who have accurate knowledge of their baby's condition will be in a better position to answer queries as to what is wrong with their baby, and how it will affect the life of the family in the future.

A disabled child can bring extended families closer together through their support for the parents and the care of the child. Friends, too, will often rally round and give practical help and moral support. But occasionally the opposite reaction is uppermost and contact with parents and their baby ceases abruptly. Some people may be embarrassed, upset or even afraid, nor knowing how to react to a disabled baby and may conclude that it is easier to stay away.

Life is never the same after the birth of any baby. With the birth of a disabled baby, this change is increased a hundredfold. Hospital and clinic visits will need to be fitted into the daily routine, special treatments or foods may need to be given or in-patient spells may be necessary. And all this on top of caring for a physically and/or learning disabled child who is not developing along the same lines as everyone else's baby. No wonder parents become quite exhausted, particularly as normal sleep patterns in the baby may be difficult to establish. Help from a variety of agencies should be made available to parents who have a baby suffering under these, and similar, conditions.

Accurate **diagnosis** is one of the most important first-line aspects. Following on from this, information can be given as to what the future holds. This can take up much time, as parents will need to go away to think about the implications for their future lives. During this time many potential day-to-day problems will occur to them. So once again, an important part of helping parents to come to terms with their baby's disability is allowing time – maybe again and again – for discussion. Worries and fears need to be voiced so that explanations can be given, together with information on various agencies that can offer practical help.

Social workers will need to be involved with the family from the early days. Advice on help available, be it financial or local respite care facilities, for example, can do much to relieve the isolation felt by parents.

Respite care facilities will become more necessary as time goes by. Here, families closely vetted for suitability volunteer to look after a disabled child in their own home for a given period of time. This may be for a weekend only, or for a two-week break. This allows the parents of the disabled child – and also any other children in the family – to go perhaps to a wedding or other family celebration or to enjoy a holiday without the continual worry of the care of a disabled member. The 'host' family receive payment for their input into the care of the child. People who offer respite care facilities are frequently themselves working in the field of disability, and so are well used to caring for disabled children. Parents can thus be sure that their child is receiving the best possible care whilst they are away.

This brief break from the continual care can do much to relieve the exhaustion of the parents. It is important for the couple to have the chance to be together for some time to pursue common interests which are impossible to indulge with a disabled child – for example, walking or a visit to the theatre. This aspect is probably of greater importance in today's society than a generation or two ago. Few parents today have the support of an extended family who will share the burden of care of children.

Self-help groups, of which a number have been formed over the past decade, certainly in the UK and USA, can also provide much support. It is good to be able to write, meet or telephone a family who have a child with a similar syndrome. Day-to-day management of problems can be talked over in an informal manner. Many of these self-help groups also provide useful material on the specific condition as well as arranging meetings for members. Many of these self-help groups are registered charities which organize fund-raising activities for research. These groups, together with social worker input, give valuable information regarding various items of equipment available for disabled living.

Contact-a-Family (CaF) is a charitable organization which correlates the work of self-help groups. As well as supplying a directory of self-help groups (kept up-to-date for subscribers on a twice yearly basis), this organization has a number of other functions:

- advice is given to over 800 local parents groups anywhere in the UK;
- there is a national telephone help line (0171 383 3555) answering queries on individual children's disabilities;
- a quarterly journal is also published, together with a range of factsheets on various related topics, such as welfare benefits, special educational needs, starting a parent's group and fund-raising;
- CaF also provides a national voice for families to improve national awareness of various disabling conditions.

If any of the self-help group addresses and telephone numbers in this book are unavailable for any reason, CaF will give the relevant addresses and telephone numbers. CaF can be contacted at:

170 Tottenham Court Road
London W1P 0HA
Tel. 0171 383 3555
Fax. 0171 383 0259

Professionals caring for a child with a disability on a regular basis will find the CaF directory of value. Parents can be given information on local groups who can do much, by way of support and practical help, to ease the trauma of learning that a much-loved child has a 'syndrome'.

It is important that every disabled child has his/her abilities, both physical and mental, **assessed** regularly on an on-going basis. This can be done at a hospital, a clinic specializing in assessment of abilities or at the child's own doctor's surgery if he/she is particularly interested in such problems.

If the parents are contemplating a further pregnancy, **genetic counselling** is important after the birth of a disabled child. The exact diagnosis of the disabling condition will need to be known, and a family tree of other possibly similarly disabled members will need to be drawn up. There are a number of genetic counselling centres in the UK where such advice can be given (their addresses are given at the end of this book). Any future pregnancy must be monitored carefully, making techniques such as ultrasonic scanning, chorionic villus sampling and amniocentesis available to the parents.

Finally, **bereavement counselling** may be necessary at a later date. Many children with specific disabling conditions cannot look forward to a normal lifespan. In a number of syndromes, death can occur in the late teenage years or early twenties. Even though they have been led to expect this, the actual event is a shattering blow to the parents. Used to a busy life caring for their disabled child, suddenly their days seem long and empty. Feelings of relief are mixed with the inevitable feelings of sadness and loss. This again can lead to an excess of the guilt normally felt after a death: 'Perhaps there could have been more done for our child?', 'Perhaps we were not as dedicated as we should have been?' and most pertinent of all in a genetically acquired condition, 'Was it our fault?'. Parents will need much sympathetic support over the weeks and months following the death of a disabled child.

All is not gloom, however, following the birth of a child with an inherited disability. Families can be brought closer together in the care of their child. Pleasure can also result from helping with the everyday successes of life with a disability. Many families will be certain that their quality of life is enhanced by their disabled child with his/her own unique personality.

As our knowledge of the causes and effects of disability increases, the more help can be given to members of our society – all over the world.

Achondroplasia

ALTERNATIVE NAME

Chondro-dystrophy.

INCIDENCE

The incidence of achondroplasia is thought to be around one in every 25 000 births. There are between 25 and 30 babies born with achondroplasia every year in the UK. The mode of inheritance would suggest this figure is variable, due to the inability to predict new mutations, which can also result in achondroplasia. Both sexes can be affected, and it is possible to diagnose achondroplasia at birth. A number of achondroplastic pregnancies are known to miscarry, or the baby dies in the early weeks of life, particularly if the birth has been premature.

HISTORY

There are quite a large number of conditions and syndromes in which short stature is a prominent feature. Achondroplasia is unique in that the limbs are short, whilst the trunk is of a normal size. This is obvious at birth. The short stature of other conditions will only become obvious as the child matures.

Many achondroplastic men and women used to be the 'small people' working in circuses. This was the only occupation open to them until comparatively recently when enlightenment regarding suitable careers became the norm. Achondroplasia is now no bar to many jobs and professions, including medicine and teaching.

CAUSATION

The mode of inheritance is two-fold. Achondroplasia can be inherited as an autosomal dominant characteristic or can arise as a new mutation. It is thought that the latter accounts for most of the babies born with achondroplasia. It has been suggested that advanced paternal age may be a factor, but this has not been proved. The basic fault is that the epiphyseal plates of the limbs fail to produce adequate cartilage tissue. This starts before birth.

CHARACTERISTICS

Skeletal effects

Short stature: this is of a very particular type. The arms and legs are short, whilst the trunk and head are of normal size. Specialist charts are currently being produced to monitor the growth of achondroplastic children. The usual charts will not give a true picture of whether the child is growing satisfactorily or not, due to the disproportion in the body configuration in an achondroplastic child.

Head size gives rise to the appearance of being out of proportion to the trunk. There are a number of reasons for this. Head circumference is on the upper limits of normal and also achondroplastic children usually have a broad, prominent forehead with often a larger than normal lower jaw. The bridge of the nose is also often flattened, and this adds to the optical illusion of a top-heavy head. In contrast to this, the base of the skull and the foramen magnum are small. This latter fact can sometimes cause compression of the spinal cord in this region, giving rise to respiratory problems. Some achondroplastic children have died suddenly and unexpectedly from this cause. Hydrocephalus, due to the abnormalities of the foramen magnum at the base of the skull, occurs in a few children with achondroplasia. This, too, will add to the disproportionate size of the head.

The **pelvis**, if X-rays are taken, also has abnormal features. The roof of the hip joint is flat with a protruding bony spike. This can account, in part, for the unusual waddling gait of many people with achondroplasia. The fact of having very short legs also makes for an unusual walking pattern – especially when trying to keep up with long-legged companions!

The normal curves of the **spine** are accentuated. The lower lumbar curve is more marked than usual. This has little effect during childhood, but can give rise to lower back pain later in life.

Eventual **height** rarely reaches more than 55 in (140 cm).

Hands are broad and short, the lack of length being in the shortness of the metacarpals (from wrist to knuckles). Fingers in contrast are of normal length. The achondroplastic child cannot close his/her fingers together; they remain widely spaced in spite of all his/her efforts to approximate them.

Children with achondroplasia are often **hypotonic**. Due to this, they are often late in sitting and starting to walk. It is inadvisable to put too much pressure on them to hurry these skills along, as the combination of weak muscles and a large head puts a great strain on the spine with the probable effect of increasing the lordosis in the lumbar region. **Mental abilities** fall within the normal range and intellectual abilities can be high. Psychologically, most achondroplastic children are well adjusted to their small size. But occasionally problems with body image can occur.

Ears: frequent middle ear infections are common. Later, a conductive deafness can occur, due to the repeated ear infections. Sensori-neural deafness can also occur.

MANAGEMENT IMPLICATIONS

These revolve largely around the short stature and its associated problems.

Short stature: problems with this aspect of achondroplasia will increase as the child matures. During infancy and the toddler years, lack of height is not too noticeable, but around the early school years it becomes obvious when the achondroplastic child stands alongside his/her peers. Orthopaedic treatment to lengthen limbs has been available in recent years. Much thought by the child and the family will be needed before embarking upon this long treatment, but much confidence can be gained by the child when several inches can be added to height. Growth hormone has been given at appropriate times during the growing years, but recently strong doubts have arisen about this treatment as it may have severe effects on the child later in life.

Practical aids, such as suitable seating, low shelves for storage of personal possessions, smaller sports equipment and general low-level living devices can make the life of the achondroplastic child easier. From the teenage years on, difficulties with ticket machines, high steps onto buses and trains as well as driving problems – to mention just a few – must all be appreciated and help given wherever possible.

Emotional effects, both on the affected child and the family, must not be forgotten. Parents of normal height can become greatly distressed by their child's difficulties, and where the inheritance is obvious, the parent also affected can suffer from guilt reactions. Sensitive counselling of the whole family, with time to think through all the implications of short stature in particular, should be available. Care must also be taken to ensure that the child with achondroplasia is not treated as younger than his/her chronological age. It is all too easy to forget that in all aspects of development other than height, the child is exactly the same as his peers, with similar needs – and, of course, potentially with similar behaviour. (Clearly this applies equally to all children of short stature.)

Orthopaedic abnormalities can result from abnormalities in the spine. 'Slipped discs' in the lower lumbar region are not uncommon in later life, and must be appropriately treated, probably by surgery. Leg lengthening operations and operations to correct excessively bowed legs can be undertaken in selected cases, and will do much to improve the quality of life. Watch must be kept for spinal cord compression weakness and tingling in lower limbs – due to the abnormality in the region of the foramen magnum. Most importantly, breathing patterns must be watched carefully during childhood.

Hearing: the frequent attacks of otitis media must be treated quickly and adequately. Hearing assessment following attacks of infection should also be carried out to determine if hearing has been affected by the infective process. Myringotomy may need to be performed to counteract conductive deafness.

THE FUTURE

Sufferers from achondroplasia have a normal life span, and are generally healthy individuals, as long as spinal abnormalities are not severe. Symptoms of cord compression (for example, weakness, pain or tingling in arms or legs) must be investigated and treated urgently. Job prospects are limited only by the lack of height, as intellectual ability should not be affected. With recent advances in surgery to increase height, public awareness and less discrimination in the workplace, job prospects show even more promise.

Achondroplasia is no bar to conception and pregnancy, although the delivery of the baby will need to be by caesarian section due to the pelvic abnormalities in most cases. Genetic counselling is advisable before embarking on a planned pregnancy. There is a 50% chance of the condition being inherited if one parent is achondroplastic and a 75% chance if both parents have the bone disorder.

(**Hypochondroplasia**. This is a modified form of achondroplasia in which only a certain part of the condition is present. In children with this disorder it is the upper parts of both arms and legs which are disproportionately short – the remainder of the body and limbs being of normal size and proportions.

Short stature is also a feature of this condition, but will not be as marked as in achondroplasia.

Final height is rarely more than 65 inches (165 cm).

Inheritance patterns are the same as for achondroplasia, with a 50%

chance of the child having the condition if one parent has hypochondroplasia.)

SELF-HELP GROUPS

Bone Dysplasia Group (part of Child Growth Foundation)
2 Mayfield Avenue
London W4 lPW
(Tel. 0181 994 7625; 0181 995 0257)

This is a network of families offering advice on problems associated with achondroplasia and other conditions with lack of normal bone growth.

Disabled Living Foundation
346 Kensington High Street
London W14 8NS

Equipment for the Disabled
2 Foredown Drive
Portslade
Sussex BW4 2BB

Aicardi's syndrome

INCIDENCE

The incidence of Aicardi's syndrome is not known. But as the definitive triad of signs are recognized this syndrome may not be as rare as was originally supposed. Only girls are affected due to the mode of inheritance, and all races seem to be involved. Certain criteria for a diagnosis of Aicardi's syndrome have recently been described. Similar signs and symptoms occur in other conditions, and it is probable that these, at times, are confused with true Aicardi's syndrome sufferers.

HISTORY

In the late 1960s, Dr Aicardi described in the French literature a recognizable set of signs and symptoms now known as Aicardi's syndrome. By 1980, over 100 patients had been identified. In 1982, the genetic basis for the syndrome was reported.

CAUSATION

At the present state of knowledge, Aicardi's syndrome seems to arise due to chromosomal abnormality of the X chromosome. It is probable that most usually this abnormality occurs as a new mutation, as there has only been one reported family with two children with the same condition. Only girls are affected as the condition seems to be incompatible with life in the male foetus. At present, antenatal diagnosis is not possible.

CHARACTERISTICS

Infantile spasms are one of the invariable characteristics of Aicardi's syndrome. These are convulsions of a specific type which begin in early infancy. Many of these fits can occur during the course of the day and are sometimes known as 'infantile spasms' or 'salaam attacks' due to the position taken by the baby during a convulsion – rather like a formal bow. 'Hypsarrhythmia' is another name. This type of convulsion continues to occur in Aicardi's syndrome throughout life in a modified form. These continual fits are very damaging to brain function, occurring as they do with such frequency.

The EEG features of Aicardi's syndrome are unusual and quite unique. There is obvious independent activity of the two halves of the brain on the tracing. It has been suggested that this may be due, in part, to the absence or gross abnormality of a specific part of the brain – the corpus callosum.

Eye abnormalities: the whole eye is often small. But the particular abnormality of the eye in Aicardi's syndrome is the appearance of the retina. When viewed with an ophthalmoscope, a number of 'punched out' areas are seen in this vital part of the eye. With this appearance blindness would seem to be inevitable, but this is not always so, although vision must of necessity be restricted. Nevertheless, sufferers frequently do become blind as they get older.

Brain abnormalities can be seen on CT scanning and magnetic resonance imaging. A specific area of the brain – the corpus callosum (that part of the brain linking the two cerebral hemispheres together) – are affected. This feature results in severe **developmental delay** and **learning disability**. All aspects of development are affected, both large and fine movements as well as speech. The restricted vision also adds to the problems of fine movements.

These are the three major problem areas which are to be found in all sufferers from Aicardi's syndrome. Other abnormalities are also commonly seen, but are not always present.

The **spinal column** often shows fused vertebrae or only partially developed vertebrae. As a result of this **scoliosis** frequently occurs, giving rise to respiratory problems due to restricted breathing movements. This problem is made worse by ribs often being misshapen or sometimes absent altogether. So the whole function of the chest – both heart and lungs – is under stress.

Deformities of the **hands** can also be present. The size of the baby's **head** can be small and does not show the usual continuing growth. The head circumference (a routine measurement in all babies, used to indicate brain development) is frequently on the lower line of the centile charts.

MANAGEMENT IMPLICATIONS

Convulsions: these are especially difficult to control. Some sufferers have had to be prescribed as many as seven different anti-convulsants to control the seizures. ACTH has been used to good effect, particularly when given in the early months. It is thought that early control of convulsions, as far as is possible, may help to reduce further brain dysfunction.

Visual problems: the exact extent of the visual loss is difficult to diagnose accurately, due both to the anatomical effects in the retina and to the learning disability found in Aicardi's syndrome children. Little help can be given due to the patchy loss of retinal tissue – this latter being vital for normal vision.

Developmental delay and **learning disability** are profound and will need full-time skilled help as the child matures. Few children with Aicardi's syndrome develop any speech. Walking is usually achieved, but can be very late in occurring. Self-help skills, such as feeding and dressing, will be only slowly, if ever, achieved. Schools for profoundly disabled pupils will be necessary. Respite care in order that parents can have a break from caring for their disabled child should be made available if at all possible. It is important that other children in the family should be able to have an active holiday without the restrictions necessary for the care of their disabled brother or sister.

Children with Aicardi's syndrome do seem to be especially prone to coughs and colds. These infections can often extend to their lower respiratory tract giving rise to bronchitis or pneumonia. The relative immobility of the child is not helpful in preventing these complications.

THE FUTURE

This is bleak for sufferers from Aicardi's syndrome. Full-time care will need to be given throughout life. Control of seizures will also be a life-long problem, and many children succumb to respiratory tract infections.

The description of Aicardi's syndrome being of such recent origin, there are no substantiated reports as to how long these children can be expected to live. The oldest known survivor was 15 years old in 1989.

SELF-HELP GROUP

Recently a self-help group, known as CORPAL, has been formed. This includes families with children who have agenesis of the corpus callosum with no additional problems. The effects of this latter disorder are very variable, ranging from completely normal development to severe disability. The address to contact is:

CORPAL
7 Bromley Avenue
Flixton
Manchester M31 3HZ
(Tel. 0161 748 0014)

Aims and provisions: support and information for families; international links; promotion of research.

Albinism

INCIDENCE

Albinism is a rare condition. There are a number of variants in which individuals are affected differently. Many affected people have an altered lifestyle due to their albinism. It is thought to occur in approximately one in 200 000 people overall. Albinism occurs in all races, being more common in some peoples than others. For example, the incidence in France is one in 100 000, whilst the incidence in the San Blas Indians of Panama is seven in 1000.

There are a number of other syndromes which have albinism as part of their characteristics.

HISTORY

Albinos, the name by which people with albinism are frequently known, have been recognized for centuries. The name was originally applied by the Portuguese to white African negroes.

The name is also applied to animals and plants lacking pigment.

CAUSATION

Albinism is a genetically inherited disease, most forms being transmitted in an autosomal recessive manner. The basic fault is one of an inborn error of metabolism, the enzyme tyrosinase being defective. So melanin, the pigment giving eye, hair and skin colour, is not available. This is in spite of there being normal numbers of pigment-forming cells (melanocytes) in the basal layer of the skin. But due to defective tyrosinase activity, these cells are not able to produce melanin.

There are several different types of albinism, which can be difficult to distinguish clinically. In one type there may be some pigmented naevi on the body, and the hair in coloured peoples may be yellow instead of white. This would suggest that in this particular type there is some tyrosinase activity.

Albinism may also be partial, so that the full effects of a complete lack of melanin are not seen. Very blond children with fine, delicate skin which burns easily on exposure to the sun probably have a minimal form of albinism. A type of albinism can be part of the clinical pattern of two further syndromes – Waardenburg's syndrome, which is associated with deafness and Chediak–Higashi syndrome, which also has blood and immunological problems associated with the condition. Eyes alone can be affected (ocular albinism) and this type is thought to be inherited in an X-linked manner.

Antenatal diagnosis is only possible by biopsy of the foetal skin, which is rarely performed.

CHARACTERISTICS

Skin: albinos have a very fair skin which, without the protection of the necessary melanin, burns very readily in sunlight. Along with this fair skin goes white, silky hair. Eyebrows, eyelashes and other body hair is also white.

Eyes: the iris is a very pale pink or blue. The redness of the retina can sometimes be seen through this translucent iris. As a result of this, photophobia (dislike of light) is common. Abnormalities in the visual pathways are always present in true albinism. Defective antenatal development of optic fibres and poor formation of part of the retina due to lack of pigment is the basic problem. This leads to much reduced vision. **Nystagmus** – rapid backwards and forwards movement of the eyes – can also be present. Strangely enough, nystagmus does not interfere too much with vision, although some children develop an unusual head posture in an effort to compensate for the flickering of their eyes. Nystagmus in those albinos who show it usually improves with advancing years. Squints can also be present, although not invariably so.

MANAGEMENT IMPLICATIONS

Skin: very great care needs to be taken with albino children in sunlight. Even dull days, with the sun behind cloud, can cause burning if the skin is exposed. Cover-up clothes are essential at all times and adequate sunscreen creams are also advisable. In hot sunny countries the problems can be acute.

Eyes: vision must be checked on a regular basis and corrective lenses prescribed as far as is possible. It is especially important that school-age children should receive annual visual checks. Vision can deteriorate rapidly during periods of rapid growth in all children, and albino children are especially at risk. It is frequently not possible to obtain perfect vision, due to the eyes' developmental abnormality which is always present in complete albinism. Vision does not deteriorate any more than normal with age. Dark glasses are often necessary to protect the eyes from light due to the lack of protective pigment in the iris. Squints, when present, should be corrected orthoptically or surgically in order to maximize all possible vision. Early correction of squints is vital if amblyopia – lack of vision in one eye – is to be avoided.

Education: about 20% of albino children will need special educational facilities due to their visual problems. These children are not blind, although their vision is such as to come within the legal definition of blindness. Emphasis in schools should be put on those activities at which the children can do well. Other children, with fewer visual problems will be able to attend mainstream schools, but with care always being taken regarding their sensitive skins.

THE FUTURE

Albinism does not restrict life span. However, career prospects can be limited. Work outside in all weathers has to be avoided due to the skin problems.

Restricted distance vision in many cases will give rise to problems of obtaining a driving licence. Near vision, however, is usually good, so careers needing fine, close work are most suitable, especially as these kind of skills also involve working indoors, avoiding skin problems. Children with normally pigmented skin can be born to a couple who both have albinism. Genetic counselling should be given due to the number of variants of the condition. Careful scrutiny of family trees, ancestors with very pale skins and fair hair and maybe other abnormalities will give clues as to possible inheritance patterns.

Skin cancers can arise more readily due to the lack of protective melanin. So any patch of skin which shows signs of permanent reddening, soreness or excess itching should receive immediate attention.

SELF-HELP GROUP

Albino Fellowship
16 Neward Crescent
Prestwick
Ayrshire KA9 2JB
(Tel. 01292 70336)

Aims and provisions: support and fellowship; leaflets on special problems.

Albright's syndrome

ALTERNATIVE NAMES

Albright's hereditary osteodystrophy (AHO); pseudohypoparathyroidism.

INCIDENCE

Albright's syndrome is a rare condition. The exact number of children affected is unknown, but nevertheless the condition is well documented. Basically this syndrome arises from a fault in calcium and phosphate metabolism in the body which in turn is due to faulty parathyroid hormone activity. Both boys and girls can be affected, but with girls more commonly seen with the syndrome.

The biochemical abnormality need not give rise to symptoms and can be found in totally asymptomatic and clinically normal people. The abnormality is only discovered when specific routine testing is undertaken in relatives of children who have Albright's syndrome.

HISTORY

In 1942 Albright first recognized the syndrome as being due to a failure of the action of the parathyroid hormone on calcium and phosphates in the body. Research continues and in 1980 the basic molecular defects of the disease were described.

CAUSATION

Albright's syndrome is a genetic disorder with some uncertainties still existing as to the exact mode of inheritance. It may be that the syndrome is X-linked, which would account for the higher incidence in girls. However, some authorities consider Albright's syndrome to be inherited as an autosomal dominant characteristic, but with sex modifications.

CHARACTERISTICS

Albright's syndrome may not be recognised until mid-childhood, although convulsions due to the altered calcium and phosphate levels can occur in infancy, when the diagnosis can be made. The following characteristics are found in the complete syndrome in mid-childhood.

Short stature: this is not usually as marked as in many other syndromes (cf Turner's syndrome). Body proportions are normal with legs and arms in keeping with the rest of the body (cf achondroplasia). Most people with Albright's syndrome reach a final height of around 60 inches (152 cm) which is quite an acceptable height for most activities.

Obesity occurs commonly and makes the lack of height appear more obvious. Typically, Albright's children have plump, round faces with a short neck. This tendency to excessive weight gain can also be noted before birth, so that many babies with Albright's syndrome have a high birth weight. Weight gain is also rapid in the first few months. (Whilst the above picture of height and weight is usual in Albright's syndrome, these measurements can still be within the normal range.)

Skeletal system: due to the abnormalities in calcium and phosphate metabolism, unusual calcification can occur in parts of the skeleton. For example, hips and pelvis can have abnormal bony configurations as well as limb bones.

Short fourth and fifth fingers are a fairly constant finding and can help in confirming the diagnosis. The shortness of these fingers is very specific, and is due to the relative shortness of the terminal phalanges of these digits.

Eyes: cataracts can occur in Albright's syndrome, although this is not an invariable finding.

Learning disability: intelligence is sometimes normal in children with Albright's syndrome but the usual range of intelligence quotient is between 20 and 99, with a mean level of 60. The level of intelligence would seem to depend upon blood levels of calcium and phosphate. Those children with low levels are likely to have a higher degree of disability than those with normal levels of these chemicals.

Thyroid underactivity is more commonly found in children with Albright's syndrome than in the general population. It is important that this is diagnosed early if present, so that treatment with thyroid hormone can be given. It is thought probable that early treatment of this problem reduces the incidence of possible learning disability.

MANAGEMENT IMPLICATIONS

Hypocalcaemia: if low levels of blood calcium are found, treatment with vitamin D has been found to be effective. Calcium supplements may also be necessary, as may other drugs to reduce the amount of calcium excreted.

Hypothyroidism must be treated with replacement thyroid hormone if levels of this hormone are found to be low. Signs of hypothyroidism, such as weight gain, slow speech, a hoarse voice, scanty hair and dry skin should be watched for in a child known to have Albright's syndrome. Blood levels can then confirm the clinical diagnosis of hypothyroidism.

Dietary measures to reduce obesity should be undertaken (and kept up!). The help of a dietitian should be enlisted as it is important that nutrition is adequate for proper growth and development. Dietitians, too, have a wealth of skills which make eating the right foods fun rather than restrictive. Overweight children can suffer miseries at school. As well as being the target for teasing, they find it difficult to join in physical activities, and are often the last person to be asked to join a team. From the health point of view, excess weight puts unwanted strain on growing joints. There may also be a link with hypertension in later life. So all efforts should be made to keep weight gain to a minimum.

Learning disability, if present, may need special schooling and extra help later in childhood. Routine developmental checks and later, school performance tests, will determine if there are any problems. Children of normal intelligence with Albright's syndrome are perfectly able to cope with mainstream schooling. Care must be taken, however, that dietary regimes and any necessary medication are strictly controlled.

Eyes: cataracts will need ophthalmic assessment and treatment if present. Routine visual tests should be done to detect problems early. Good lighting and some form of magnification can be helpful before any necessary operative procedures are undertaken.

Genetic counselling must be offered when the reproductive years are reached.

THE FUTURE

A normal lifespan is to be expected in those with Albright's syndrome. However, watch should be kept on blood pressure during adult years as severe hypertension is found in over half of the adults with this condition. This finding can predispose to early 'strokes' and/or coronary thrombosis. Treatment should be given to maintain blood pressure within normal limits as far as possible. Weight control will lessen the risks of hypertension. In pregnant women with this condition, delivery by caesarian section is frequently necessary due to the bony abnormalities in the pelvis.

SELF-HELP GROUP

There is no specific group, but support and information on facilities are available from:

Research Trust for Metabolic Diseases in Children (RTMDC)
Golden Gates Lodge
Weston Road
Crewe
Cheshire CW1 1XN
(Tel. 01270 25022)

Alport's syndrome

ALTERNATIVE NAMES

Hereditary nephritis; Fechtner syndrome

INCIDENCE

The severity of Alport's syndrome can differ widely from individual to individual. This can be, in part, due to the way in which the disease is inherited. The type known as Fechtner syndrome (or Fechtner variant) is an example of this differing severity and mode of inheritance. Alport's syndrome has been reported from many parts of the world, but, up to 1989, there were no reported cases in black children. Depending on which inherited pattern is at work, incidence is either the same in both sexes or there is a preponderance of girls suffering from the condition.

One of the important factors in Alport's syndrome is the fact that this condition is thought to be responsible for up to one-sixth of the cases of specific renal disease. Alport's syndrome should always be suspected if a number of family members suffer both from renal disease and deafness.

CAUSATION

Alport's syndrome is inherited in an X-linked manner. Boys with the condition are usually more severely affected than girls are, although with this form of inheritance twice as many girls are thought to be affected.

The syndrome can also be inherited as an autosomal dominant characteristic. Under these circumstances equal numbers of boys and girls are affected. The Fechtner variant is inherited in this manner.

CHARACTERISTICS

All sufferers from Alport's syndrome will have **nephritis** to some degree. This is manifested by the passage of blood and/or protein in the urine. It is more usual for these signs to appear in mid-childhood, although the pathological changes in the kidneys have been present from the early days of life. Occasionally, bouts of mild **fever** occur in association with the progressive damage to the kidneys.

At the onset of the disease, kidney function is normal. However, gradually over the years this will deteriorate until, in the most severely affected, renal failure can occur during the teenage years. Under these conditions the waste products of metabolism will not be removed adequately from the body. The child will become progressively tired and listless and have a poor appetite. Thirst will be complained of and large quantities of dilute urine will be passed – maybe with a return to bed-wetting in the younger child.

In around half of the cases of Alport's syndrome, more commonly in boys, there will be a **sensori-neural deafness**. This deafness can be slowly progressive until little residual hearing remains. Any child with recognized renal disease should be carefully checked for a coexisting hearing loss. The deafness may develop as early as three to four years of age.

These two groups of symptoms are the main features of Alport's syndrome, but the following added problems can occur:

- in around 15% of children there will also be **visual** problems – the formation of cataracts being the most common of these;
- a specific type of skin complaint, known as **icthyosis**, can also occur in some children with Alport's syndrome. The skin, as the name implies, will be dry and scaly;
- there can also be a specific **blood disorder**, thrombocytopaenia, in which there is a low platelet count. This can lead to numerous small patches of bruising on the child's body;
- as the regretfully inevitable renal failure progresses the following events can occur at varying times:

  - the child will become **anaemic**. This is due both to the child's poor appetite and also to a reduction in the production of red blood cells;
  - a raised **blood pressure** can occur as a result of the disease process in the kidneys;
  - **bony changes** similar to those seen in rickets can occur. This again is primarily due to the kidney disease leading to a decreased absorption of calcium;
  - **growth** can be retarded by all these factors associated with the renal disease.

MANAGEMENT IMPLICATIONS

The most important aspect in the management of Alport's syndrome is the maintenance of renal function. Once the diagnosis has been made, regular visits to a paediatric neurologist (a paediatrician with a special interest in conditions of the renal tract) will be necessary. Clinical examination along with blood and urine tests and specialized X-rays and ultrasound examination will give clues to kidney function. Depending on the results of tests, various regimes of drugs and nutritional requirements will be needed to counteract anaemia, hypertension and the bony changes which may occur.

Dialysis of one form or another will eventually be necessary for the sufferer from Alport's syndrome. The most usual age for this treatment to become necessary is between ten and 15 years of age. The specific reasons for starting on this form of treatment will vary from child to child. Some children will need urgent treatment following on from some intercurrent infectious illness with which their kidneys cannot cope. In others, blood tests will show serious imbalances in the chemical composition of the blood which cannot be controlled by drugs or nutritional changes. There are three methods of dialysis which clear the waste products of metabolism from the body:

- **Haemodialysis** in which waste products are removed from the blood. This requires hospital admission two or three times a week;
- **Continuous peritoneal dialysis** in which waste products are removed from the peritoneal cavity of the abdomen. This method will need attention four times daily, but has the advantage that the child is able to lead a more normal daily life without the need for frequent hospital admission.
- **Continuous cycling peritoneal dialysis.** Similar principles are applied with this method of removing waste products, but the treatment is carried out once every 24 hours, at night. With this method there is less disturbance of family life than the six-hourly bag changes necessary with the former method.

Dialysis of any type needs a skilled team in a specialized renal unit to oversee the initial setting-up of the most suitable method and also to ensure continuous monitoring of progress. Life will obviously be difficult for the whole family when dialysis is an everyday necessity.

Kidney transplantation is the ultimate aim. This will, of course, relieve all need for dialysis and once the critical period for rejection of the new kidney is over, the child will be able to lead a normal life again.

Two other major problems must be considered. One is the progressive **deafness** from which children with Alport's syndrome can suffer. Regular checking of hearing is necessary, with the arrangement of specialized teaching if the deafness becomes profound. The other is **vision**, which must be checked regularly and appropriate treatment given if cataracts should be found to be developing.

Schooling may be problematical at times when frequent hospital admissions are necessary. Health and education authorities will need to liaise closely to provide the best facilities for the child.

Careers for children with Alport's syndrome will depend very much on the severity of the disease. With minimal lack of renal function (as is sometimes the case with girls with this condition) or kidney function restored by kidney transplantation, any career is possible. Deafness, if present, may of course lead to further difficulties. Good careers advice from someone conversant with all the possible problems associated with this syndrome is vital for the young person.

THE FUTURE

This will depend upon the severity of the renal disease. Boys fare worse than girls in this respect and renal failure is frequently fatal before the age of 30 years unless kidney transplantation has been successfully undertaken. Girls often have a normal life span in spite of kidney abnormalities being present.

SELF-HELP GROUPS

British Kidney Patient Association
Bordon
Hampshire GU35 9JZ
(Tel. 01420 472021)

National Kidney Federation
6 Stanley Street
Worksop
Nottinghamshire S81 7HX
(Tel. 01909 487795)

Aims and provisions: both these groups offer advice and support to families; the British Kidney Patients Association also runs holiday dialysis centres and raises money to provide financial support for families.

Angelman's syndrome

ALTERNATIVE NAME

Hitherto known as the 'happy puppet' syndrome.

INCIDENCE

The exact number of children with Angelman's syndrome is not known, but over 80 definite cases have been reported in the literature.

HISTORY

Children with Angelman's syndrome were previously referred to as suffering from the 'happy puppet' syndrome, due to the rather jerky movements seen in association with outbursts of laughter. This name has now been dropped since more knowledge has been gained regarding the genetic basis for this condition.

CAUSATION

Angelman's syndrome is a chromosomal disorder, the faulty chromosome being chromosome 15. There has been found to be a deletion in the same region of this chromosome as is seen in Prader–Willi syndrome. In spite of this, the two syndromes are very different clinically. It is thought that the problem in the case of Angelman's syndrome is derived from the maternal side, in distinction from Prader–Willi syndrome in which the defect is considered to arise from the father. Most children with this syndrome occur out of the blue, although five families have been reported to have two children with the same condition.

Angelman's syndrome is not evident at birth, but becomes obvious as the child matures. There is no antenatal test available at present. It is advisable, if possible, that parents should receive genetic counselling before embarking upon a further pregnancy.

CHARACTERISTICS

Microcephaly: at birth, the baby's head circumference is within normal limits. As the child grows, this important measurement is seen to fall behind the other parameters of growth, never reaching the normal size.

During infancy, **feeding** can be a problem, largely due to poor brain development, leading to difficulties in sucking.

Normal **sleep patterns** are also often difficult to establish. Babies with Angelman's syndrome are frequently hyperactive, and seem to need little sleep – and that little at inappropriate times!

Developmental delay leading to severe **learning disability** occurs over the early years. Babies up to approximately one year of age can appear to be progressing normally, but from then on, signs of delayed development are to be seen, in particular the following:

- **Speech** is affected to a disproportionate degree. Expressive speech is never properly attained, although receptive language develops so that children with Angelman's syndrome are able to understand simple commands.
- **Walking** is late, and a typical jerky gait in noticeable in the early years, although this does tend to improve in later childhood. Occasionally, the unusual gait produces deformities in joints, which may need correction at a later date.
- **Arm movements** are also jerky and stereotyped. (These movements, combined with the unusual gait, gave rise to the name 'happy puppet'.)
- **Hand flapping**, often associated with outbursts of inappropriate laughter is another obvious characteristic. The laughter is not thought to be connected with epilepsy – as can be the case – but rather due to involuntary motor activity.

Seizures are common during infancy and childhood and a characteristic pattern is seen on EEG tracing. These fits may decrease spontaneously in later life.

Facial features: children with Angelman's syndrome tend to have large mouths with widely spaced teeth. Tongues tend to protrude, and this is especially noticeable during the outbursts of laughter.

Children with Angelman's syndrome are usually happy and affectionate young people. One of the greatest problems associated with this syndrome is the child's inability to speak. But in spite of this disability, children appear to enjoy life.

MANAGEMENT IMPLICATIONS

Early **feeding** and **sleep** problems, with a varying degree of **hyperactivity**, will need help. Small, frequent feeds and a regular routine in an attempt to rationalize the sleeping pattern is the best method of approach. This can take much patience and support. Short-term sedation may be necessary to break the difficult sleeping pattern, and also to allow the parents to get some sleep themselves.

Speech therapy is necessary as the speech problems become obvious. Non-verbal techniques of communication such as sign language training may help to relieve some of the frustration felt by the child due to the lack of usual communication skills. It is rare that any understandable speech is ever attained.

Seizures will need to be controlled with anti-convulsants. Dosage and type of anti-convulsant will need to be checked on a regular basis as fits tend to reduce naturally later in childhood.

Learning disability will require educational facilities for severely disabled pupils, where there is an emphasis on training in self-help skills. This training will need to be continued in a suitable environment after statutory school-age has been passed.

THE FUTURE

Regrettably, children with Angelman's syndrome will never be able to lead an independent life. Full-time care will be necessary, preferably in a warm, loving environment where some degree of suitable communication can take place.

Life expectancy is thought to be normal. There have been no children reported being born to sufferers from Angelman's syndrome.

SELF-HELP GROUP

Angelman Syndrome Support Group
15 Place Crescent
Waterlooville
Portsmouth
Hampshire PO7 5UR
(Tel. 01705 264224)

Apert's syndrome

ALTERNATIVE NAMES

Acrocephalo-syndactyly type 1; Vogt cephalo-syndactyly.

INCIDENCE

Apert's syndrome is one of a group of syndromes which are characterized by premature fusion of the bones of the skull, together with malformations of the hands and feet. This type of acrocephalo-syndactyly is one of the most serious of the group. The condition is rare, only occurring in between one in 100 000 to one in 160 000 births. Both boys and girls can be affected, and the condition can be diagnosed at birth.

CAUSATION

Apert's syndrome can be inherited as autosomal dominant, but few cases of direct inheritance from either parent are known. Most of the cases seem to arise as new mutations. There have been suggestions that older fathers may be more at risk of having a child with Apert's syndrome, but this has not been conclusively proved.

CHARACTERISTICS

The bones of the skull in new-born babies are normally separated from each other. This aids the process of birth by the skull being able to mould to the birth canal. Soon after birth the edges of these flat bones become joined together by fibrous tissue in specific places. These positions of fusion are known as the 'sutures' of the skull. It is at these positions that future skull growth occurs to accommodate the underlying growing brain. In Apert's syndrome (and also in other syndromes of a similar nature) these sutures fuse together prematurely. It is this early fusion that gives rise to the typical characteristics of the head and the face seen in children with this syndrome.

Head: the most striking feature of babies born with Apert's syndrome is their high, prominent forehead, often with a marked swelling in the mid-line. The back of the head also tends to be more flattened than is usual.

Facial features: in contrast to the prominent forehead – and also often large lower jaw – the nose is small and flattened. This can give rise to both breathing and feeding difficulties in the neonatal period. **Eyes** are also large and prominent, and are usually widely set apart.

Ears tend to be low-set and a congenital hearing loss is frequently present.

The **hands** of babies with Apert's syndrome can also be malformed. The severity of this deformity can vary a good deal. Sometimes only webbing of the skin between the fingers is present, but the worst cases show some bones of the hands completely fused together, usually involving the second, third and fourth fingers. If this occurs the hands have a claw-like appearance.

Feet are usually normal, but in rare cases can have a similar appearance to the hands.

Mild **learning disability** occurs in around 50% of children with Apert's syndrome – the remaining 50% having normal intelligence. Any slowing of abilities will gradually become apparent over time and will be picked up during routine developmental checks.

Hydrocephalus, caused by faulty drainage of cerebrospinal fluid in the ventricles of the brain, is a not infrequent complication of Apert's syndrome.

A further unusual complication, seen in a large number of young people with this syndrome, is severe **acne** during the adolescent years.

MANAGEMENT IMPLICATIONS

Initially, **feeding** and **breathing** difficulties commonly occur. The nasal abnormalities make it difficult, if not impossible, for the baby to breathe whilst he/she is feeding. So in the early days, nasogastric feeding will probably be necessary. By three to four months these problems resolve themselves as the nasal passages enlarge with general growth.

If **hydrocephalus** occurs, a 'shunt' will need to be inserted to drain the excess fluid away from the brain. This complication, so often seen in Apert's syndrome babies, can be difficult to diagnose in the early stages, as the more usual signs of hydrocephalus tend to be obscured by the unusual shape of the skull. Careful checks on neurological signs, such as increased muscle tone in the lower limbs for example, and developmental patterns will be necessary to exclude this added problem.

Surgery to correct the premature fusion of the bones of the skull will need to be undertaken, and this may well mean a series of operations over the years. It is thought that these corrective procedures may help to prevent learning disability. Surgery may also be necessary on hands and sometimes feet to achieve maximum function and for cosmetic reasons.

Regular **developmental checks** are of vital importance to diagnose any slowing, or regression of physical function and other skills as early as possible.

Due to frequent stays in hospital for various necessary operative procedures, Apert's syndrome children will need extra loving stimulation between these visits so that vital learning processes are not missed out.

Understanding and support for parents and child will need to be available, due not least to the unusual facial and limb features. Other children – and regrettably also adults – can be particularly unkind to children who look 'different'.

THE FUTURE

Life expectancy for people with Apert's syndrome can be normal, but is dependent upon the degree of involvement of the central nervous system. Career prospects are limited by the degree of disability experienced due to hand deformities and also to mental abilities. Some restrictions in work possibilities may also be encountered due to the unusual facial features.

SELF-HELP GROUP

There is no specific Apert's syndrome group, but support, advice and friendship can be obtained from:

'Let's Face It' (network for the facially disfigured)
10 Wood End
Crowthorne
Berkshire RG11 6DG

This organization, which has international links, has a junior branch linking parents who have facially disfigured children.

Cranio-facial Support Group
44 Helmsdale Road
Leamington Spa
Warwickshire CV32 7DW
(Tel: 01926 334629)

Aims and provisions: support for all families with facial problems; news-letter.

Arthrogryposis

INCIDENCE

There are a number of similar conditions which all fall under the main heading of the arthrogryposes. The full name of the commonest of these is arthrogryposis multiplex congenita (AMC). Probably the next commonest sub-group is 'distal arthrogryposis' in which only the hands and feet are affected. There are a number of other variants described, all of which have similar characteristics, but show some specific features. For example, in some children there is more emphasis on weakness of the muscles, whilst others have greater problems with neurological involvement of certain spinal cord segments.

The incidence of the commonest sub-group – AMC – is around one baby in every 10 000 being born with the condition. Both boys and girls are equally affected.

CAUSATION

The arthrogryposes are genetically inherited conditions. With the wide variety of known types, the inheritance pattern cannot be generalized. Distal arthrogryposis is inherited as an autosomal dominant condition, whilst AMC is thought to arise spontaneously as a new mutation. So it is important that when genetic counselling is given the exact diagnosis is known. In this way predictions of further children being born with the abnormality can be given more accurately.

Babies with arthrogryposis can be diagnosed at birth. Hints that foetal movements may be diminished can be confirmed by ultra-sound investigations over a specific period of time, for example one hour. Delivery can sometimes be difficult due to the relative immobility of the baby due to his genetic inheritance. This traumatic delivery can, at times, lead to some degree of learning disability.

CHARACTERISTICS

The common feature that affects children with any of the arthrogryposes is **joint deformities**. It is usual that many joints are affected. In distal arthrogryposis it is only the joints of the lower legs and forearms that are affected. All of these deformities are due to the soft tissues around the joints being contracted, or stiffened. Due to this, the joints themselves are rendered almost immobile and certainly without normal useful function.

The following description is of a baby born with the severe form of the commonest of the arthrogryposes – AMC.

Joint deformities: the baby with this form of arthrogryposis will lie in a very typical position soon after birth due to the deformities to be found in his/her joints. Shoulders will be pushed forward as arms are rotated inwards with flexed wrists and fingers turned into the palms of the hands. In a similar way, feet are flexed into a position having the appearance of a 'club foot' deformity.

Muscles in many cases are small and weak, often being replaced by fibrous or fatty tissue. Without adequate muscle power, joints are made even more immobile. A very noticeable feature in some babies with AMC is the lack of normal elbow and/or knee creases, which is such an obvious feature of most new-born babies. This is directly due to the lack of muscle development.

Short stature can be a feature in later life, as normal growth of bone is, in part, dependent on adequate movement. Without normal muscle this is impossible. The shortness is not extreme, but nevertheless obvious.

Naevi: these 'strawberry' marks are very commonly seen in babies with AMC, especially in the mid-line of the face and body.

Following on from these minor abnormalities in the mid-line of the body can be the more serious ones of **defects in the abdominal wall; inguinal hernia; asymmetry of the face**. These problems fortunately only occur in relatively few babies with AMC. Specialized care and treatment will be necessary for babies with these more severe defects.

MANAGEMENT IMPLICATIONS

It is important that the diagnosis of arthrogryposis is made early on in the baby's life so that treatment to mobilize limbs as far as possible is started early.

Physiotherapy is the mainstay of treatment, and concentrates mainly on mobilizing any muscle tissue that is present. Passive stretching of affected limbs, with joints put gently through the full range of movement on a regular basis, is of great value.

Splinting of affected joints in optimum position is also necessary. This has to be done very carefully in order to avoid damage to the weakened muscular tissue. The advice of an orthopaedic surgeon, working in close liaison with the physiotherapist, is vital for future maximum function. Maximum mobility should be the aim, so that bone growth is diminished as little as possible.

Most children with arthrogryposis manage quite adequately in mainstream **schooling**. Stairs can be a problem and adaptation with ramps, for example, may be necessary if buildings are not all on one level. Physical education lessons will not be possible for all but the most minimally affected children. Other suitable activities should be arranged during these lessons for the child with arthrogryposis if full integration into mainstream schooling is to be achieved. The help of the occupational therapy department at the local hospital can do much to give advice on suitable occupations, which can also help with limb mobility.

THE FUTURE

Children with arthrogryposis can lead full, satisfying lives within the bounds of their physical limitations. Mental ability is not affected in any way by the condition, so any number of careers are open. Obviously those activities needing physical strength or mobility are not possible, but numerous other sedentary and intellectual pursuits are options. Expected lifespan is not decreased by arthrogryposis.

For women with arthrogryposis normal vaginal delivery will probably not be possible, and babies will need to be delivered by caesarian section.

SELF-HELP GROUP

The Arthrogryposis Group (TAG)
1 The Oaks
Gillingham
Dorset SP8 4SW
(Tel. 01747 822655)

Aims and provisions: support and information for affected families; research programmes; social events and annual conference; video available.

Asperger's syndrome

INCIDENCE

The incidence of Asperger's syndrome is not yet known, as no large-scale detailed studies have been carried out, although research is continuing in this direction. The most recent work seems to suggest that boys are affected around seven times more frequently than girls. This syndrome is generally referred to as occurring in those children who are amongst the more able of those suffering from autism. The classification is somewhat confused, but at the present time Asperger's syndrome refers to children with less severe autistic features. They are children who can use non-emotional speech, but who show obsessional interests and tend to be clumsy. The incidence of autism is thought to be around one in every 2500 live births, so Asperger's syndrome is but a part of this overall incidence.

HISTORY

It was in 1944 that an Austrian psychiatrist, Hans Asperger, first described the characteristics of children who showed lack of social adjustment and much self-absorption. Dr Kanner, at much the same time, also reported similar features but with more emphasis on the specific speech and language problems. Dr Lorna Wing in the UK has done much work on autism.

CAUSATION

There is no known definitive cause of autism, or of Asperger's syndrome. Other syndromes, such as the fragile X syndrome, can show autistic features to a greater or lesser degree. Dr Asperger considered that this syndrome must be genetically transmitted. He noted a higher incidence of similar characteristics in the fathers of those children with the syndrome. Some children – about half of one series – had some history of birth problems, leading to the conclusion that in some cases organic brain deficiencies may be a causative factor.

CHARACTERISTICS

In a recent seminar six features were noted to be present in sufferers from Asperger's syndrome.

- Grave difficulties with **interactive play** with peers. Children with Asperger's syndrome do not wish to socialize and are unable to form relationships with other children. They are seen as 'cold', 'immature' or 'eccentric' and so are usually left to play on their own.
- Children with Asperger's syndrome become **totally absorbed** in one specific hobby or aspect of life to the exclusion of every other facet of daily living. This interest may be anything from chess to stamp-collecting or astronomy, the subject often having a highly intellectual content.
- Children with this syndrome need to adhere strictly to **routine** in all aspects of daily living. They become extremely upset if this stereotype is upset. For example, if on holiday the usual bedtime is relaxed this one minor alteration in the timetable can be very distressing for all the family!
- **Speech and language** are often stereotyped, with a flat, monotonous, often expressively perfect, delivery. Comprehension of language appears to fall behind the normal expressive component. For example, jokes are often taken at their face value – with sometimes embarrassing consequences.
- The vast majority of children with Asperger's syndrome show varying degrees of **clumsiness**. Actions are stiff and odd postures are often taken up.
- **Facial expression and gesture** used in association with speech is frequently inappropriate or clumsy. For example, yawning or smiling at the wrong time during a conversation is typical of the child with this syndrome.

These features are, of course, very similar to those of autism with which Asperger's syndrome is closely linked.

MANAGEMENT IMPLICATIONS

It has been noted that the more able person with autism – Asperger's syndrome – usually shows an improvement with time. After the turmoils of adolescence are over, behaviour becomes more normal and acceptable. This may be due to care and teaching in specific areas, which is of great importance in children with Asperger's syndrome.

Social and communication skills: it is in this area of development that the most difficulties are experienced. Specific efforts need to be made to teach these skills, many of which are picked up automatically by the normal child. Normal social interaction is a closed book to most children with Asperger's syndrome. The normal give-and-take of socializing can be totally bemusing so that each set of situations with the appropriate response will have to be learned. This is quite possible to achieve given the liking for rote learning and stereotyped behaviour characteristic of the child with Asperger's syndrome. It is important that the child is not allowed to withdraw into himself to avoid social activities. This is counter-productive, but a very understandable way of avoiding difficult situations.

Language may be delayed and speech therapists can pinpoint the specific areas of difficulty. For example, words which are used to describe actions (verbs) are more of a mystery than words used to denote objects (nouns). It is important that teaching of language will take place alongside the teaching of social skills in familiar situations. This will help comprehension and assist in preventing stereotypical and obsessive behaviour.

Behavioural therapy: dealing with the obsessive ritualistic behaviour of children with Asperger's syndrome is one of the more difficult problems. Probably the best approach is a graded change of behaviour patterns, starting off with small steps and continuing slowly until the rituals no longer obtrude in normal life.

The difficulties in forming relationships must always be remembered in children with this condition. 'Coldness' and lack of concern for other people's thoughts and feelings will probably always be a feature of the child's personality. Account must be taken of this facet when activities and careers are being planned.

Schooling: dealing with the disabling problems caused by Asperger's syndrome is complex, needing much sensitivity to help the sufferer. Specialists with a particular interest in the syndrome can be found by contacting the support group. There is no one particular type of school suitable for all Asperger's syndrome sufferers. Some children will be able to manage in mainstream schooling, whilst others may fare better in any one of a number of specialized schools. Each child needs to be placed according to their own specific abilities.

THE FUTURE

Depending on the severity of the manifestation of Asperger's syndrome some form of employment is often possible in adult life. Work involving a regular routine is the best choice, and the sympathetic understanding of eccentricities by employers and fellow workers is important. Other more severely affected men and women, particularly those with speech and language difficulties, are unable to hold down any kind of job, so sheltered accommodation and care will be needed for life. But even in severely affected people, a reduction in disability does seem to occur with time.

SELF-HELP GROUP

Asperger Support Network is part of:

The National Autistic Society
276 Willesden Lane
London NW2 5RB
(Tel. 0181 451 1114)

Aims and provisions: support and information; contact with local groups; schools and centres managed for adolescents and adults; courses and conferences; research activities.

Ataxia-telangiectasia

ALTERNATIVE NAMES

Louis–Barr syndrome; Boder–Sedgwick syndrome.

INCIDENCE

Ataxia-telangiectasia is a very rare condition, affecting only between one baby in every 30 000 to 50 000. There is a comparatively high number of cases in some countries, Turkey being quoted as one of these. This is possibly due to the fact that intermarriage between close relatives is more common. Both boys and girls can be equally affected.

CAUSATION

Ataxia-telangiectasia is thought to be transmitted as an autosomal recessive characteristic. This would account for the high incidence in countries where it is more likely that parents are related. There may be further cases where there is no direct link, the condition being due to a new mutation. Recently, gene mapping has demonstrated that the ataxia-telangiectasia is located on chromosome 11.

Antenatal testing is difficult at present, and modes of inheritance strongly depend on looking at other members of the family in detail. Serum alpha-fetoprotein levels are frequently raised in people with ataxia-telangiectasia, but not invariably so. This fact can help with diagnosis.

Ataxia-telangiectasia is not apparent at birth and only becomes obvious between the ages of one and two, when the child starts to walk.

CHARACTERISTICS

Walking: As soon as a definite walking pattern is established it is noticeable that the toddler is more unsteady on his/her feet than would be expected at the developmental stage reached. This is quite apparent after the age when tumbles are the norm for the new walker. This ataxia persists throughout life and, regrettably, tends to worsen as the child matures. Later, involuntary movements of limbs become apparent, much as seen in certain types of cerebral palsy. (In ataxia-telangiectasia the basic pathology is a very much reduced number of specialised (Purkinje) cells in the cerebellum; that part of the brain associated with the control of balance. As with many disorders there may be an enzyme defect involved.)

Speech can become slurred and disjointed, again due to the difficulty of control of muscular movement. But after the initial period of deterioration in the pre-school years, this particular problem should stabilize, and the child with ataxia-telangiectasia can always make him/herself understood.

Prominent blood-vessels, **telangiectases**, appear later on the white part of the eyes. Little dilated vessels are seen to be coursing over the eye, rather as if the child had conjunctivitis without the surrounding inflammation seen in this infective condition. Unlike conjunctivitis, the eyes are not sore or itchy. Characteristic changes similar to those seen in the eye can also sometimes be seen on the ears.

Infections of all kinds are frequent and even minor ones can be serious. This is due to an associated defect in the immune system of the child with ataxia-telangiectasia. Respiratory infections, which can be difficult to treat adequately, are the most common.

Malignancies, at any site in the body, are more common than usual. It is thought that around one-third of all ataxia-telangiectasia sufferers will develop cancer at some time in their lives.

Sensitivity to radiation is a further feature of ataxia-telangiectasia. This becomes of vital importance when radiation is needed to treat any cancerous growths that occur. Fibrous tissue, as a result of scarring due to the radiation, almost always results even with the carefully controlled doses given to treat malignant growths. (Normal X-ray examination – for example, necessary to diagnose the exact nature of a respiratory infection – is not harmful, as the dosage is low.)

Slowing of **growth** can occur in some children with ataxia-telangiectasia, but this does not always occur.

Sexual maturity is often late in being attained. In girls, this is due to lack of ovarian growth and, therefore, of function.

MANAGEMENT IMPLICATIONS

Although there is no specific treatment which can halt the course of the disease, there is much that can be done to make life easier for ataxia-telangiectasia sufferers and their families.

The ataxia can occasionally be helped by prescribing anti-spasmodic drugs. But the on-going nature of the situation must eventually be appreciated and a suitable lifestyle organized.

Most children will be confined to a wheelchair by the time they are ten years old and schooling has to be geared to this. A school for physically disabled pupils may be needed if buildings in local mainstream schools are not suitable – for example, a lack of ramps and suitable toilet facilities.

Typewriters or wordprocessors are useful if the ataxia affects hands and arms, making writing illegible. Special guards can be fitted making it easier for the child to hit the correct keys.

Speech therapy can be helpful in the early years to assist with the proper development of this skill. This can do much to help communication problems.

Infections must be reduced to a minimum as far as is possible. For example, relatives and friends should be asked to stay away from the child if they think they are incubating a respiratory tract infection. It is a practical impossibility to avoid all infection in children, but these must be treated quickly and adequately by the appropriate antibiotic.

The early stages of **cancer** must be watched for and any suspicious symptoms investigated fully and quickly. In particular, any low-grade fever continuing for any length of time must be viewed seriously. This may be due to a hidden source of infection or early manifestation of cancerous growth. Following on from this, special care with radiation therapy must be taken if cancer does occur, due to the high sensitivity of ataxia-telangiectasia sufferers to this form of treatment.

THE FUTURE

Life expectancy for the child with ataxia-telangiectasia is not great, and many will die in their twenties or thirties. Overwhelming infection or the results of malignant disease account for most of these tragically early deaths.

SELF-HELP GROUP

Ataxia-telangiectasia Society
42 Parkside Gardens
Wollaton
Nottingham NG8 2PQ
(Tel. 01602 287025)

Aims and provisions: support and contact with families; information by leaflet and meetings.

Batten's disease

ALTERNATIVE NAMES

Batten–Vogt syndrome; Kuf's disease (adult form).

INCIDENCE

Batten's disease is one of a large group of diseases which have a metabolic basis for the signs and symptoms seen. There are over 1000 of these metabolic conditions described. They all have in common some enzyme malfunction which results in imbalances of chemicals in the body. Signs and symptoms will be wide-ranging depending on which system of the body is most involved. The substances involved in Batten's disease (and related conditions) are the neuronal ceroid-lipo-fuscinoses (NCL). Batten's disease has at least four main types, the age of onset of the symptoms being the main differentiating point. It is a comparatively rare condition, although an incidence of one in 13 000 of the infantile type has been reported in Finland. Both boys and girls can be equally affected.

HISTORY

Many of the metabolic disorders have been known and described for years. It is only fairly recently, however, that the biochemical basis for many of these conditions has been understood. With increasing knowledge more groups of signs and symptoms (syndromes!) are being found to be due to an enzyme malfunction.

CAUSATION

Batten's disease is inherited as an autosomal recessive characteristic. The gene is located on chromosome 16, and antenatal diagnosis is possible by amniocentesis. Genetic counselling for future pregnancies is advisable.

CHARACTERISTICS

The four different types of Batten's disease are all characterized by progressive mental and physical deterioration, loss of vision and convulsions. Each of these aspects has a different emphasis in the different types.

Infantile type (also known as the Santavouri or Finnish type)

This type becomes obvious at around one year of age. **Convulsions** occur at this time and a fall-off in **mental development** is noticed. The normal development abilities slow, and the 'milestones' tested by routine developmental checks fall behind the norm. The ability to walk, instead of gradually increasing in strength and stability, becomes more and more unsteady.

Head circumference (that excellent indicator of brain growth in the early years) fails to increase along the normal growth lines as plotted on growth charts and microcephaly becomes obvious within a year or two.

Regrettably, the course of the disease is rapidly downhill, and death usually occurs between the ages of five and six years, most often due to some intercurrent infection.

Late infantile type (also known as Jansky–Bielchowsky type)

Development proceeds normally until two to four years of age. At around this time, **convulsions** occur, and become more and more difficult to control.

The child's **walking** becomes increasingly clumsy and ataxic and fine motor movements are also affected. Many of the skills already learned in both these areas of development become increasingly difficult to perform.

Along with these problems goes an increasing **visual loss**. This is due to a degeneration of the retina, again as a direct result of the enzyme defect. Nothing can be done to halt this process and the child will eventually lose most of his/her vision.

Mental deterioration also occurs and skills previously learned are lost.

As with the infantile form, death occurs in childhood, usually by ten years of age and, again an intercurrent infection is the commonest cause.

Juvenile NCL (also known as Speilmeyer-Vogt disease)

This type does not make its presence known until between six and ten years of age. The first signs of this form of Batten's disease is a diminution in vision. This is due to changes in the pigment of the retina. As a result of this the ability to transmit images to the brain is lost.

Within a few months of this deterioration, there is a slowing of **mental abilities. Convulsions** also occur as with the other forms of Batten's disease with earlier onset.

Again, muscular co-ordination problems occur, walking becomes ataxic and fine hand movements become clumsy and difficult to perform.

Paralysis can be the final outcome and death occurs between the ages of 15 and 25 years.

Adult type (also known as Kufs' disease)

The signs can begin as early as puberty – around 13 to 15 years of age or may not become obvious until the late twenties.

The most marked effects initially in this type are the **personality changes** seen. The young person's behaviour may become unpredictable with outbursts of laughing or crying and other bizarre episodes. Manic phases can be especially difficult to handle and respite care is valuable for parents during this time. (It can, of course, be difficult to differentiate between this behaviour and the often incomprehensible behaviour of normal adolescence! But in adult Batten's disease, the personality changes are progressive and can end in severe dementia.)

Later, problems of **balance** resulting in an ataxic gait are seen.

In marked contradistinction to the earlier forms of Batten's disease, visual disturbances are not usually seen. Convulsions are also not a feature.

People with this condition can survive into middle-age.

MANAGEMENT IMPLICATIONS

Control of **convulsions** is one of the mainstays of medical treatment. However, this can be difficult, and often many different anti-convulsant drugs (or combinations) will need to be tried. Sometimes anti-Parkinsonian drugs can be of value in helping the ataxic symptoms.

Support for the family of the child with one of the types of Batten's disease is of great importance. Once the diagnosis has been firmly made, parents should be counselled as to the course and final outcome of their child's condition. A sympathetic, knowledgeable ear should be available whenever necessary, if at all possible, to answer queries. This is especially important where there is more than one member of the family affected by Batten's disease.

Respite care may need to be arranged (particularly during an especially difficult phase, perhaps with manic behaviour to cope with). Parents and other children in the family will need to be able to take a holiday without a disabled member to worry about. Contact with institutions for the blind can also be helpful to give advice on aids for failing vision.

Schooling for the older child with Batten's disease will probably need to be in a special centre as the disease progresses. Continuous assessment of mental abilities, as well as frequent checks on the state of the child's vision, will need to be done to provide the most suitable environment.

Recently, bone-marrow transplantation in selected children has been undertaken in an attempt to halt the disease.

THE FUTURE

This is bleak for children with the forms of Batten's disease which have an early onset, as death occurs before the age of ten years. The forms arising later also have an unhappy outlook with declining mental abilities, as well as visual problems in the juvenile type. As with all disability, children are happiest and best cared for in a warm, loving family environment. The backing of respite care is of importance in supporting families.

SELF-HELP GROUP

There is no specific self-help group, but the following organization gives help, information and advice for all metabolic diseases affecting children:

Research Trust for Metabolic Diseases in Children (RTMDC)
Golden Gates Lodge
Weston Road
Crewe
Cheshire CW1 1XN
(Tel. 01270 250221)

Beckwith–Wiedeman syndrome

ALTERNATIVE NAMES

Beckwith syndrome; EMG syndrome.

INCIDENCE

The actual incidence of Beckwith–Wiedeman syndrome is not entirely clear, but it has been suggested that seven in 100 000 births is a probable figure. It is thought that there are a number of children with the syndrome who have not been diagnosed. Some babies born with an abnormality around the umbilicus probably also have Beckwith–Wiedeman syndrome, or at least a variant of the condition.

A much higher incidence in the West Indies has been reported – one baby in every 13 700 being the figure quoted. Both boys and girls are affected.

HISTORY

It was in 1963–64 that Dr Beckwith in America and Dr Wiedeman in France reported independently on babies with a set of specific characteristics. Since this time, much has been reported and written on this condition.

CAUSATION

Beckwith–Wiedeman syndrome is a genetic disorder. The exact mode of inheritance is nor clear at present, but it is probable that the syndrome is inherited as an autosomal dominant. The syndrome is also thought to arise sporadically as a new mutation.

In 1980 ultra-sonic examination found evidence of the specific characteristics of the Beckwith–Wiedeman baby at the 20th week of pregnancy. These abnormalities found include the defective umbilicus and the enlarged kidneys.

CHARACTERISTICS

Umbilical abnormalities are seen at birth in babies with Beckwith–Wiedeman syndrome. These can range from a small umbilical hernia to a complete failure of the muscles of the anterior abdominal wall to close together. This latter severe defect will need urgent surgical repair to protect the abdominal organs which will only be covered by thin membranous tissue. (This defect is known as omphalocele.)

The **tongue** in babies with this syndrome is unusually large and protrudes from his/her mouth. This can give rise to breathing problems as the enlarged tongue can fall back into the throat and impede breathing.

As the child matures, further problems can occur with tooth eruption, and some children with this syndrome are unable to close their top and bottom front teeth together – an 'open bite'. (It has been suggested that the hydramnios that frequently accompanies pregnancies with a Beckwith-Wiedeman baby is due, in part, to the inability of the foetus to swallow amniotic fluid because of the enlarged tongue.)

Birth weight is usually above average with Beckwith–Wiedeman babies. During the first few months of life the baby puts on weight rapidly. Growth, both height and weight, is usually along the 90th centile on the standard growth charts. On X-ray examination an advanced bone age is seen throughout childhood. Along with this unusual gain in weight and height goes an increased rate of growth of certain organs of the body, most usually the kidneys. The adrenals – those endocrine organs sitting on top of each kidney – are also frequently enlarged. Also occasionally there is an excessive overgrowth of a particular part of the body – maybe one limb only or the whole of one side of the body. This excessive growth rate slows after the first few years.

Hypoglycaemia (low blood sugar) in the very early days of life occurs in a significant number of babies. Symptoms of hypoglycaemia include convulsions, breathing and feeding problems, lethargy and cyanosis. All these symptoms could be due to a number of conditions, but if the possible relationship between hypoglycaemia and Beckwith–Wiedeman syndrome is recognized, the diagnosis can be made early. It is important that this hypoglycaemia should be treated early as it is a well-known factor in the causation of later learning disability. The hypoglycaemia is thought to be due to the overgrowth of insulin-producing cells in the pancreas.

Facial characteristics: children with Beckwith–Wiedeman syndrome tend to have small noses with rather prominent brows. At birth, and for the first year of life, flame-like naevi are often seen over the eyelids and forehead.

Ears, in many cases, have been reported to have a slight indentation either on one lobe, or on both. This is just one further clue to diagnosis.

Tumours of the kidney (Wilm's tumours) or of the adrenal cortex are more likely to occur in children with this syndrome. This is probably an anomaly of the increased growth pattern seen in so many children with the Beckwith-Wiedeman syndrome.

MANAGEMENT IMPLICATIONS

Umbilical abnormalities must be treated surgically with a degree of urgency if they are severe. Infection and injury are ever-present threats where the defect in the abdominal wall is large. A small umbilical hernia can, of course, be left until the baby is more mature and better able to withstand operative procedures.

Neonatal hypoglycaemia must be diagnosed and treated in order to prevent future learning disability.

The enlarged **tongue** usually becomes less of a problem as the surround-ing structures of the child's face grows. Orthodontic treatment for unusual 'bite' patterns may be needed later in childhood. A large, soft teat is an advantage when feeding the baby who has Beckwith–Wiedeman syndrome. In very rare cases the tongue enlargement persists so that breathing during sleep is a problem. The organ can fall back and block respiratory passages. Under these circumstances, operative procedure to reduce the size of the tongue may be necessary. Physiotherapy advice is to put the baby to sleep on his side. This will aid respiration.

Speech therapy may occasionally be necessary to overcome the relative clumsiness of the tongue.

Watch must be kept for **tumours**, in particular Wilm's tumours, through-out childhood. Very often the first intimation of the presence of this tumour is a swelling felt in the abdomen. Surgical removal and postoperat-ive treatment will be necessary in these circumstances.

THE FUTURE

Children with Beckwith–Wiedeman syndrome should expect a normal lifespan, as long as malignancies do not occur. Any career is open to them as long as neonatal hypoglycaemia has been dealt with satisfactorily, preventing reduction of mental abilities.

Genetic counselling before pregnancy is advisable.

SELF-HELP GROUP

Beckwith–Wiedeman Group
The Drum and Monkey
Hazelbury Bryan
Sturminster Newton
Dorset DT10 2EE
(Tel. 01258 817593)

Charcot–Marie–Tooth disease

ALTERNATIVE NAMES

Peroneal muscular atrophy.

INCIDENCE

The incidence of Charcot–Marie–Tooth disease is undetermined, but it is estimated that around 130 000 Europeans are affected. There are a number of variations of Charcot–Marie–Tooth disease in which deafness and kidney disease are more apparent, and these variations are thought probably to be more common than Charcot–Marie–Tooth without these aspects. Boys and girls can be equally affected.

HISTORY

Charcot–Marie–Tooth disease is one of the most well-known of a group of familial diseases which have as their main symptom muscle weakness, mainly in the lower limbs. The cause of this weakness is a degenerative process in the nerves supplying the muscles. There are very many causes of this neuropathy, including other inherited diseases, for example Friedrich's ataxia, deficiency conditions such as diabetes and vitamin deficiencies, infective conditions such as shingles and the effects of various toxins – for example, botulism and certain drugs. Care must be taken that these causes are eliminated before a diagnosis of Charcot–Marie–Tooth disease is made. In recent years the genetic basis of the familial neuropathies has been established.

CAUSATION

Charcot–Marie–Tooth disease is inherited as an autosomal dominant. The severity of the symptoms can vary markedly in different individuals, with some aspects being more in evidence in some people than in others.

A few families have shown direct male to male inheritance. Recent reports have noted that a duplication of part of chromosome 17 seems to be responsible for Charcot–Marie–Tooth disease.

CHARACTERISTICS

Symptoms of Charcot–Marie–Tooth disease do not arise until the child is around ten years of age, or maybe a little younger.

Legs and feet: Charcot–Marie–Tooth disease first shows itself in the lower limbs. The child's gait will become awkward and he/she will not be able to keep up with his/her peers when speed is required. The muscles running down the front of the lower leg are the ones primarily affected. The thigh muscles are rarely involved in the muscle wasting which eventually becomes apparent in the lower leg, when the legs characteristically assume a 'stork-like' appearance. Ultimately, foot-drop becomes obvious with toes being dragged along as each step is taken. Fortunately, children with this condition rarely 'go off their feet' altogether and walking, although slow can be maintained. Toes will become fixed later in a claw-like position due to the muscle wasting. Cramp and tingling sensations also occur at a relatively early stage.

Fingers and arms: the upper limbs can be affected in a similar way, usually to a milder degree and the onset is later. The pathology of these effects is basically one of de-myelination of the peripheral nerves, those supplying the muscles of the limbs, and giving rise to the characteristic symptoms of muscular weakness and eventually deformity.

Hearing: a sensori-neural loss often becomes evident in later life. The first signs of deafness can occur in the teenage years and by early middle-age the deafness is frequently severe.

Renal effects – nephritis – can very occasionally be part of the symptomatology of Charcot–Marie–Tooth disease. If this does occur, it is usually around the late twenties that symptoms first begin to appear.

MANAGEMENT IMPLICATIONS

These are largely ones of **mobility** in childhood. Early years are frequently quite normal apart from this point of view – the child walking, running and climbing along with his/her peers. It is when the child is seen to be having difficulties with sports and other physical activities in the school years that carers should be alerted to possible problems. He/she may also be complaining of cramping pains in his/her legs. The diagnosis becomes obvious when muscle wasting and footdrop occurs. Children with Charcot–Marie–Tooth disease should not be encouraged too strongly to take part in physical activities, but rather encouraged to pursue other interests which do not need too much physical input.

Advice and treatment from an orthopaedic surgeon and a physiotherapist regarding foot-drop will help to prolong activity. Specially designed ankle or foot orthoses are a valuable aid in combatting the footdrop. These can be conveniently worn under socks so that the child will not feel too different from his/her peers.

Hearing: the gradual loss of hearing which is a common feature of Charcot–Marie–Tooth disease must be monitored on a regular basis and hearing aids must be fitted when the hearing loss makes normal communication difficult.

THE FUTURE

Life expectancy is not limited by Charcot–Marie–Tooth disease. The main problems encountered will be ones of mobility and increasing deafness. Suitable careers must be chosen bearing in mind the possible on-going problems associated with this condition.

A watch must also be kept in early adult life for signs of renal problems which can occur at this time in sufferers from this condition.

SELF-HELP GROUP

Charcot–Marie–Tooth International (UK)
121 Lavernock Road
Penarth
South Glamorgan CF64 3QC
(Tel. 01222 709537)

Aims and provisions: support, information and advice to members; raises money for research.

CHARGE association

ALTERNATIVE NAMES

CHARGE syndrome; choanal atresia.

INCIDENCE

This is a recently described condition, and only a few cases, around 50, are known at present. An 'association' rather than 'syndrome' was thought to be a more appropriate name for this condition, as the cause has not been isolated as yet. The name CHARGE is an acronym of the main features seen. For a definite diagnosis to be made, at least two of the major features must be present. About twice as many boys as girls have so far been found to be affected.

HISTORY

In 1979, Dr Hall first noticed the occurrence of other specific signs in association with the nasal defect of **choanal atresia**. (Choanal atresia is a life-threatening condition in which either one or both of the baby's nostrils are blocked by a bony or membranous defect. As all babies breathe entirely through their noses, it is vital that this type of blockage should be noted and treated urgently.) In 1981, it was decided that CHARGE was an appropriate acronym for this set of symptoms.

In 1986, Dr Davenport suggested that the condition should be termed a 'syndrome' rather than an 'association' of defects, as there was probably a common aetiology for all the features seen. Both names are used now.

CAUSATION

This has not as yet been clarified. Most cases seem to be isolated, but both autosomal dominant and recessive modes of inheritance have been described. Family histories, as the number of babies suffering from these defects are known, will help solve this problem.

CHARACTERISTICS

CHARGE is an acronym for Colomba of the eye; Heart disease; choanal Atresia; Retarded growth; Genital hypoplasia; Ear abnormalities.

Colomba of the eye is a defect in which parts of one, or a number of, the structures of the eye are missing. For example, there may be a 'gap' in the iris or a similar defect in the retina or other vital structures of the back of the eye. These latter are obviously of greater import than a defect in the iris, as vision will be directly affected. Eyelids can also be affected in a similar manner. The whole eye may also be smaller than normal. Effects on vision vary according to the type of defect present. About 80% of people with the CHARGE association show this feature.

Heart defects are variable and range from complicated problems, such as Fallot's tetralogy, to a patent ductus arteriosus or a ventricular septal defect. Any baby born with choanal atresia must be examined carefully for signs of a heart defect as the two conditions occur together so frequently. Again, the effects will depend on the type and the severity of the abnormality.

Choanal atresia was the first consistent sign to be noted in this collection of abnormalities. Sometimes only one nostril will be affected by the atresia and under these circumstances the symptoms will be less severe. In fact, it may not be until the child has his/her first upper respiratory tract infection that the condition may be noticed. Here, there will be discharge of mucus from only one nostril with an unusual amount of obstruction noticed on the other side of the nose. In a severe bilateral case, however, it is vital that surgical treatment is undertaken early to repair the defect in order to prevent potentially lethal respiratory problems. With the less serious unilateral atresia, surgery can be elective at a time when the child is more mature.

Retarded growth occurs in around 80% of babies with the CHARGE association. Birth weight and length are usually normal, but by six months of age growth has slowed, in both these parameters, so much so that only the third centile on standardized growth charts is reached. Subsequent growth continues along this lower line.

Genital hypoplasia of one kind or another is also found in children with the CHARGE association. The commonest in boys is a small penis. No-one with this condition has given birth to children.

Ear abnormalities are not always present and there are a wide variety of features. The ears may have a characteristic triangular shape or may be extremely small. Hearing can also be affected, and deafness ranges from a mild loss to a profound one. Both conductive and sensori-neural losses are seen.

These are the main features of the CHARGE association, at least two of which must be present before a definite 'label' can be attached. There are also a number of other features which have been noted to be present in a high proportion of children with the CHARGE association. These include **learning disability**, ranging from mild to severe and **facial features**, which are sometimes seen, including a small lower jaw and/or a cleft lip or palate.

MANAGEMENT IMPLICATIONS

The **choanal atresia** must be surgically corrected as a matter of urgency if it is bilateral. Following this, respiratory function will be normal.

Heart defects must be looked for in all babies with choanal atresia, and treated appropriately if present.

The **cleft lip/palate** will need surgical repair at some stage during the early years if present.

Vision must be checked in early childhood if any of the other features of the CHARGE association are present. Although colomba of the iris is one of the more obvious features, it must be remembered that similar abnormalities can occur in other less visible parts of the eye.

Hearing problems should also be fully investigated and dealt with as far as possible, if they exist. Hearing aids may be necessary for some children. If the deafness is found to be present at an early age, intensive speech and language therapy will be necessary in order not to miss out on the critical age for language acquisition.

Due to the frequency of learning disability which occurs in association with the CHARGE condition, routine developmental checks must be especially carefully done at the appropriate times. Resulting from this monitoring, help can be given early for any delay in specific, or general, areas of development.

When the time comes, **schooling** needs to be geared to the child's abilities, although most will manage adequately in mainstream schools. Extra help may be needed at specific times in different areas for some children. The impact of hearing and visual problems as well as hospitalization, for cardiac problems for example, must also be remembered when schooling is being considered.

Occasionally, a specific **growth defect** has been found in children with the CHARGE association. If this is so, replacement therapy can aid growth. **Genetic counselling** is advisable if further pregnancies are considered.

THE FUTURE

The choanal atresia and the heart problems are the two most serious features of the CHARGE association. If these are dealt with adequately, a normal lifespan is to be expected. Hearing, vision and mild learning disability can all make a difference to the choice of a career and the effects of these problems must be considered.

SELF-HELP GROUP

There is no specific group associated with the CHARGE association, but the following group has recently been formed to give advice and support to children and their parents with the specific eye problems that can occur.

Colomba Support Group
43 Dinam Road
Caergeiliog
Holyhead
Gwynedd LL65 3ND
(Tel. 01407 741413)

Aims and provisions: contact with other similarly affected families; support and information by letter.

Christmas disease

ALTERNATIVE NAMES

Haemophilia B; Factor 9 deficiency.

INCIDENCE

Christmas disease is one of the bleeding disorders of which haemophilia A is the most well known. For proper clotting of the blood following injury a number of 'factors' are necessary. In Christmas disease the 'factor' that is deficient is 'factor 9'. (Haemophilia A is deficient in 'factor 8'.)

The incidence is one in every 50 000 live male births worldwide, but in the UK this figure is thought to be as high as one in every 30 000 live male births (only boys are affected, due to the mode of inheritance).

HISTORY

It was not until the early 1960s that specific treatment was available for any of the diseases associated with bleeding disorders. Until this time, much disability was suffered as a result of bleeding into the joints and soft tissues of the body following trauma even of a mild degree. Then, with the advent of concentrates of the necessary clotting factors available for use after injury, this picture changed dramatically.

In recent years, as a result of contamination of blood products with HIV infection, many tragedies have occurred with a not inconsiderable number of haemophiliac patients contracting AIDS. Heat treatment of the products used to treat haemophilia has now prevented the transmission of this vicious infection.

CAUSATION

Christmas disease is inherited as an X-linked characteristic. The condition is passed down the female line, who suffer no ill-effects, to 50% of their sons.

Antenatal diagnosis can be made by fetoscopy. Measurement of the 'factor 9' coagulation level at birth in a male baby who has a family history of a bleeding disorder will also give a diagnosis.

CHARACTERISTICS

As with haemophilia A, sufferers can be severely, moderately or only mildly affected by Christmas disease. The degree of severity depends on the actual amount of factor 9 that is present in the blood. Severely affected boys will have less than 1% of normal activity of factor 9, whilst a mild sufferer can have as much as 20% of normally-acting factor 9.

Boys with the severest manifestation of the condition will suffer **bleeding into the joints** following the slightest injury. A bang on the knee or elbow, for example, which would normally hardly be noticed, will produce bleeding into the joint with very obvious swelling and pain. Great care must be taken with children with haemophilia when they are learning to walk. Everyday tumbles on to knees in particular will produce painful bleeding into these joints. Unless adequate treatment is given, these repeated, inevitable knocks of everyday life will cause damage to, and eventual destruction of, the joint. Much deformity, pain and disability used to be the inevitable lot of haemophilia (of whatever type) sufferers.

Bleeding can also occur into the soft tissues of the body and bruising is a frequent event following only mild trauma. This easy bruising must be recognized and taken into account when there are fears of child abuse.

Minor surgical procedures, such as **tonsillectomy** or **dental extractions** for example, can lead to severe bleeding unless prophylactic treatment is given.

Infection with **hepatitis B** is a very real threat to boys with any of the bleeding disorders. This illness, characterized by general malaise, fever, lack of appetite and jaundice, can lead to serious and potentially fatal liver problems. Any boy with one of the bleeding disorders should be immunized against hepatitis B as soon as the diagnosis is made.

Treatment: the specific concentrate containing factor 9 must be used to treat haemorrhages as soon as possible after they have occurred. Parents can be given a supply to use promptly after their son has sustained an injury. This substance should also be given prophylactically before any surgical procedures are undertaken. Some boys may develop a type of immunity ('inhibitor') to their treatment. If this should happen, referral to a specialist haemophiliac centre should be made.

MANAGEMENT IMPLICATIONS

As with haemophilia A, a balance between over-protection and complete freedom must be decided upon by parents. The severity of their son's condition will obviously have a bearing on his activities. Contact sports and activities where there is a high potential for injury should be avoided. Mountaineering and canoeing are but two popular leisure activities which immediately come to mind as unsuitable for the boy with a bleeding disorder. The boy's interests should be channelled into less active but equally interesting hobbies.

Schooling should be possible in the mainstream setting. Teachers should be informed of their pupil's problems, and be aware of the action to be taken if an injury should be sustained. To cope with the possibility of the boy's parents being unavailable if such an event should occur, the telephone number of the haemophiliac centre overseeing the boy's treatment should be made available at school. Career advice must be geared towards choices which will be possible in the future for the boy with Christmas disease. Sedentary occupations with minimal physical content, and hence minimum injury potential, should be chosen.

Care should be taken when giving pain relieving drugs to haemophiliac boys. Aspirin, and similar drugs which affect platelet (an important constituent in the blood intimately concerned with the clotting process) function, should be avoided.

THE FUTURE

With prompt treatment of haemorrhage, the possibility of long-term disability has vastly improved and a useful, fulfilling life can be lived whilst suffering from Christmas disease. Obviously care will have to be continued throughout life and certain careers and leisure opportunities will not be open to these boys.

The only other possible problems connected with the disease are the possibilities of chronic hepatitis or infection with HIV. But with immunization against hepatitis B and heat-treated blood products, these problems are reduced to a minimum.

SELF-HELP GROUP

The Haemophilia Society
123 Westminster Bridge Road
London SE1 7HR
(Tel. 0171 928 2020)

Aims and provisions: advice and support for sufferers and their families.

Cockayne syndrome

INCIDENCE

Cockayne syndrome is very rare, but is well-documented in the literature. The syndrome has been reported in the USA and Japan as well as Europe. Boys and girls are equally affected. (There is a sub-group known as Cockayne syndrome type 2 in which the age of onset is much earlier. Boys are three times as likely to be affected as girls with this subgroup.)

CAUSATION

Cockayne syndrome is inherited as an autosomal recessive condition. It is thought that an enzyme defect is the basic fault. The deficient enzyme, or enzymes, are those responsible for the repair of cells following exposure to sunlight. The relationship between these effects and the other neurological problems are unclear at present. Amniocentesis at 16 weeks can determine the syndrome antenatally.

CHARACTERISTICS

The baby with Cockayne syndrome is normal at birth. All aspects of growth and development appear to be proceeding normally until between six and 12 months of age. The following characteristics then make their appearance.

Growth is drastically reduced after the initial period of normal growth. All routine measurements – height, weight and head circumference – are seen to be falling away when plotted on the normal growth charts. Severe dwarfism is the final result. Subcutaneous fat and tissue is also lost, resulting in a wizened appearance, rather like that seen in extreme old age. By four years of age this is very obvious.

Learning disability: along with the restriction in physical growth goes a fall-off in mental abilities which, regrettably, is progressive. Pathologically, there is atrophy of the actual brain tissue and de-myelination of all nerves is seen. These factors account for the progressive loss of skills.

Skin: there is severe sensitivity to sunlight in the majority of children with Cockayne syndrome. A scaly, red rash develops after only minimal exposure to sunlight. This is followed by crusting and eventually scarring together with excessive pigmentation of the affected areas. These effects are a direct result of the failure to repair damaged cells, which is in turn is due to the enzyme abnormality.

Eyes: cataracts and retinal atrophy frequently occur with increasing age, so blindness is a very real possibility.

Ears: a sensori-neural deafness is also common.

MANAGEMENT IMPLICATIONS

Learning disability: the severe progressive loss of skills, both mental and physical, seen in a child with Cockayne syndrome is devastating for the parents. Continuing sensitive counselling is necessary to help parents through this time. Eventually the child will need full-time care. Incontinence and mobility difficulties as well as visual and auditory defects all add to the disability. If the child is cared for at home, respite care to allow parents and other members of the family to have a holiday is a necessity.

Skin: great care must be taken to avoid exposure to sunlight. Cover-up clothing, including hats with brims to protect the face as well as strict avoidance of really bright sunlight altogether must be the order of the day. Protective clothing needs to be worn even on overcast days. High-factor sun-screen cream can also be applied.

Vision and hearing: deficits in these senses will need to be checked on regularly as far as is possible. Little can be done to prevent the progressive visual and hearing losses, so carers must remember the gradual loss of these methods of communication and attempt to use other methods of contact with the progressively disabled child.

THE FUTURE

Many children with Cockayne syndrome die in early childhood, but the late teens can be reached. Disability becomes profound, and full-time care will be needed.

SELF-HELP GROUP

Cockayne Syndrome Contact Group
18 Edenway
Brickhill
Bedford MK41 7EP
(Tel. 01234 270417)

This group is under the umbrella of:

Research Trust for Metabolic Diseases in Children (RTMDC)
Golden Gates Lodge
Weston Road
Crewe
Cheshire CW1 1XN
(Tel. 01270 250221)

Coffin–Lowry syndrome

ALTERNATIVE NAME

Coffin syndrome.

INCIDENCE

This was thought to be a rare syndrome, but now appears to be more common than the number of published cases suggests. Both boys and girls can be affected and the syndrome has been reported in many countries in Europe, Asia and Africa.

HISTORY

The syndrome was described by Dr Coffin in 1966 and by Dr Lowry in 1971.

CAUSATION

The Coffin–Lowry syndrome is an X-linked recessive condition. Family studies have shown inheritance to be strongly linked through the female line. Sporadic cases due to new mutations are thought also to occur frequently.

CHARACTERISTICS

Learning disability: this aspect of the Coffin–Lowry syndrome appears to be worse in boys than in girls. Most boys with the condition are severely disabled. Girls can be similarly affected, but more frequently have only mild disability or have completely normal intellectual function.

Short stature is not excessive, but most children with the Coffin–Lowry syndrome grow along the third centile of the growth charts for height. Final height is rarely more than 5 feet (152 cm). During adolescence, scoliosis and kyphosis commonly occurs, which adds to the apparent shortness of stature. Puberty occurs at the usual time.

Facial features: foreheads are square with the eyes set widely apart and a short nose. The mouth tends to be large with a full lower lip and a small lower jaw. Features often become coarsened with age.

Fingers are a very characteristic shape, being both puffy and tapering towards the tips. An excess of soft tissue accounts for the puffy appearance. Fingers are also often hyperextendible due to laxity of the ligaments surrounding the joints. (In some children, this laxity also extends to other joints of the body.)

Deafness can also be a problem, although this is by no means invariable.

Seizures can occur but, again, not every child with the Coffin–Lowry syndrome has this feature.

MANAGEMENT IMPLICATIONS

Learning disability: management of this aspect of the Coffin–Lowry syndrome will be dependent on the degree of disability found in the individual child. Serial developmental testing throughout childhood is of importance so that educational facilities can be tailored to ensure that full potential of every child is reached.

Boys with this syndrome rarely achieve normal speech. Speech therapy is helpful in evaluating the level of language attained and giving help with greater fluency and language acquisition.

Scoliosis and/or **kyphosis**: adolescence is the time when a close watch for these vertebral abnormalities is necessary. Referral for an orthopaedic surgeon's opinion, and possible treatment, is advisable for all but the mildest abnormalities. The chest deformity which can result from the vertebral problems can also give rise to respiratory effects. Early orthopaedic intervention can largely prevent this.

Deafness should be remembered as a possibility in children with the Coffin–Lowry syndrome and hearing should be tested at regular intervals.

Seizures, if present, must be controlled with appropriate anti-convulsants.

THE FUTURE

Life expectancy appears to be limited to around 40 years. Death usually occurs from cardiac or respiratory problems, often as a result of the spinal defects so commonly seen.

Boys will need special educational facilities. Girls may also require special teaching, but this is less often necessary, as they frequently have normal intellectual abilities and can successfully pursue normal careers.

SELF-HELP GROUP

Coffin–Lowry Support Group
23 Harcourt Road
Copnor
Portsmouth
Hampshire PO1 5RQ
(Tel. 01705 610226)

Cornelia de Lange syndrome

ALTERNATIVE NAMES

De Lange syndrome; Brachmann Lange syndrome; Amsterdam dwarfism.

INCIDENCE

It is estimated that one in every 10 000 babies born alive will be affected by this syndrome. Boys and girls are equally affected.

HISTORY

Cornelia de Lange syndrome was first published as a clinical entity in 1933. Dr Brachmann had previously described the condition in 1916.

CAUSATION

The cause of this serious condition still remains a mystery. Some children with the Cornelia de Lange syndrome have chromosomal abnormalities, but these are not consistently confined to one chromosome. Two research programmes – one in the UK and one in the USA – are currently in progress to determine the aetiology of this syndrome.

Some of the specific abnormalities associated with the syndrome can be detected on ultra-sonic scanning. Apart from this there is no antenatal diagnostic test available at present. Cornelia de Lange syndrome is obvious at birth.

CHARACTERISTICS

Learning disabilty is inevitably present in the Cornelia de Lange syndrome and can vary in degree from moderate to severe disability. All aspects of development are delayed. Speech is especially late and may be absent altogether.

Skeletal system: birth weight is frequently low even though a full-term pregnancy has been reached. Children are short and have a reduced head circumference (microcephaly). Noses are small and tip-tilted so that nostrils are very obvious.

Arms: there are often severe abnormalities ranging from tiny hands with a single palmar crease to partial absence of the upper limbs in some cases.

Legs are generally normal and fully formed, but there is often webbing of the second and third toes.

Babies with Cornelia de Lange syndrome are floppy at birth, and tend to remain **hypotonic** throughout their lives.

Heart defects also commonly occur, and may be of any type – no specific abnormality is typical.

Convulsions occur in many children with the Cornelia de Lange syndrome.

Excess hair is frequently seen all over the body. The eyebrows are especially bushy and often meet in the mid-line over the bridge of the nose.

Infections of all kinds can cause problems throughout life as Cornelia de Lange children seem to have a very much reduced resistance to all types.

MANAGEMENT IMPLICATIONS

During infancy, **feeding** and **breathing** problems are common, due both to the low birth weight and to the microcephaly. Babies will frequently need to be nursed in an incubator and fed by nasogastric tube for the first few weeks of life.

Convulsions need to be treated with anti-convulsant drugs. Several of these drugs, or a combinations of drugs, may need to be tried before satisfactory control is achieved.

Infections will need brisk treatment with antibiotics throughout life, due to the increased susceptibility to all types of everyday infections.

Any **heart defect** will need assessment, regular monitoring and/or treatment with drugs or surgery as necessary.

Intellectual abilities will also need to be carefully and regularly assessed. It has been found that Cornelia de Lange children respond very readily to care and stimulation of all kinds. All babies need to be spoken to on a regular basis from an early age. This and other stimuli, will ensure that each child reaches his or her full genetic potential. This aspect of child care is especially important if there is any degree of learning disability.

Schooling will require 'special education' placement as appropriate locally. Cornelia de Lange children will thrive best in a warm, loving family environment.

Children with severe **upper limb deformities** will need help from a rehabilitation centre which specializes in artificial limbs. Special equipment may be necessary for some children to maximize their abilities.

THE FUTURE

An independent lifestyle is not possible and few people with this syndrome reach old age. Their increased susceptibility to infection and long-term consequences of possible heart defects make for serious life-threatening problems.

SELF-HELP GROUP

Cornelia de Lange Foundation
'Tall Trees'
106 Lodge Lane
Grays
Essex RM16 2UL
(Tel. 01375 376439)

Aims and provisions: dissemination of information; telephone support and regional meetings; books, reports and videos are prepared by the US group.

Advice on suitable equipment is available from:

Disabled Living Foundation
246 Kensington High Street
London W14 8NS

Cri–du–chat syndrome

ALTERNATIVE NAMES

Chromosome 5 short-arm deletion; Lejeune syndrome.

INCIDENCE

It is thought that up to 1% of all profoundly disabled children suffer from this syndrome. Until genetic studies became available this syndrome was not classified, although the very typical cry during infancy had been noted.

The exact incidence is not known, but is probably about one live birth in 20 000. The sexes appear to be affected equally, although it has been suggested that cri–du–chat syndrome is more common in girls.

HISTORY

Professor Lejeune fully documented this syndrome in the 1960s.

CAUSATION

Cri–du–chat syndrome is a chromosomal disorder. The chromosome affected is chromosome 5; the short arm of this chromosome being deleted in children affected by this syndrome. Most cases arise as a new mutation, although a balanced translocation may be present in one or other of the parents. Under this latter circumstance there is an increased risk of recurrence in a future pregnancy. The age of either parent appears to have no bearing on the advent of the syndrome. Antenatal diagnosis can be made by chorionic villus sampling at nine to 12 weeks of pregnancy and later (16 weeks) by amniocentesis.

CHARACTERISTICS

A **weak high-pitched cry** is the most obvious characteristic of the cri–du–chat syndrome. This cry is very like that of a kitten – hence the name of the syndrome. The reason for this typical cry is the relatively small size of the larynx. As this structure enlarges with growth, the unusual cat-like cry is lost.

Short stature: birth weight of babies with cri–du–chat syndrome is usually on the low side of average. Throughout life, children with this syndrome are small, rarely growing to a height above that measured on the third centile of the standard growth charts.

Facial characteristics: 98% of cri–du–chat children are microcephalic. Head circumference is small at birth, and continues to grow only slowly. Children with this syndrome have round faces with a downward slant to the eyes, which are widely set apart. There is often also a divergent squint present.

Congenital heart disease is a relatively common occurrence in children with cri–du–chat syndrome. Around 30% have this problem, the defect most usually being a patent ductus arteriosus. The murmur of this abnormality can usually be heard at birth. Symptoms of heart disease will depend on severity of the defect.

Learning disability is always severe and there are no reports of children having an IQ of above 35. Evidence of this disability can be suspected in the early months of life when the 'milestones' of smiling, following objects visually and later reaching out for toys are absent or much delayed. As development proceeds the disability, regrettably, becomes more and more obvious.

Poor muscle tone: the baby with cri–du–chat syndrome is floppy at birth and can experience severe breathing difficulties. Head control is slow in being attained, and movements are restricted. Most adults with the condition have poor muscle development.

MANAGEMENT IMPLICATIONS

During infancy, there are severe **respiratory** and **feeding** difficulties. This is due both to the small size of the larynx and associated structures and also to the general floppiness of the baby. The baby may initially need nursing in an incubator to promote adequate respiration. Tubefeeding may also be necessary for proper nutrition. Even if the baby can suck adequately, feeding is very slow, which in turn exhausts the hypotonic baby. Respiratory problems improve with the growth in size of the respiratory passages over the succeeding months.

Congenital heart disease may need surgical repair depending on the site and size of the defect, and the effects this exerts on the baby's cardiac function. Obviously the baby's general condition will need to be carefully assessed and steps to improve both nutritional and respiratory functions taken before any surgery is contemplated.

Learning disability: it has been specifically noted that early and frequent stimulation of the baby with cri–du–chat syndrome is beneficial. So, verbal stimulation – talking all the time to the baby whilst attending to his/her needs – as well as other auditory and visual stimuli are important in developing all possible mental abilities. Only very few children with this syndrome develop any communication skills at all. But with sufficient, appropriate stimuli some responses and feedback from the child can be gained – albeit at a very primitive level.

Children with cri–du–chat syndrome, in common with all other children, are happiest and reach their maximum potential if they can be brought up in the warmth and security of their own homes, or alternatively in a secure, stable environment with plenty of one-to-one contact. If home care is possible – and this is a hard task for any family – respite care facilities should be made available. This will enable parents, and any other children in the family, to have a holiday without the constant worry of a severely disabled member.

Walking skills are usually attained late. This is due both to the hypotonia seen in infancy and also to the degree of learning disability. Structured exercise from a physiotherapist may be helpful and benefit the poor muscle development.

Squints, if present, may need correction both from a cosmetic point of view and also to ensure that maximum visual input can be received – of even greater importance in a disabled child than a child who can adapt more readily. Amblyopia can develop all too quickly in an untreated squinting eye.

THE FUTURE

The child with cri–du–chat syndrome will regrettably never be able to lead an independent life and will always need full-time care. Life span is limited, mainly due to respiratory and/or cardiac problems, but many children survive into adulthood. The oldest recorded adult with cri–du–chat syndrome is 56 years of age.

SELF-HELP GROUPS

Cri–du–chat Syndrome Support Group
43 East Trinity Road
Edinburgh EH5 3DC
(Tel. 0131 552 1806)

Aims and provisions: support through personal contact; information on the condition.

Another group which gives help and advice to children with learning disabilities and their parents is:

MENCAP
123 Golden Lane
London EC1Y ORT
(Tel. 0171 454 0454)

Crouzon's syndrome

ALTERNATIVE NAME

Cranio-facial dystosis.

INCIDENCE

The exact incidence of Crouzon's syndrome is unknown, but it is a rare condition. However, the incidence of similar conditions which also have abnormalities of the head and face are not uncommon. A figure of one in every 2000 children with such abnormalities has been quoted. There are many syndromes associated with this type of disfigurement, examples being Pfeiffer's syndrome, Apert's syndrome and Carpenter's syndrome. Boys and girls are affected in equal numbers. The condition can be recognized at birth by the unusual facial features and is confirmed by X-ray examination. There is no antenatal diagnosis possible at present.

CAUSATION

Crouzon's syndrome can be inherited as an autosomal dominant condition. In these circumstances there is a wide variety in the physical expression of the disease – some cases being more severe than others.

In around 50% of cases, however, the condition appears as a fresh mutation. Some authorities consider these sporadic occurrences of Crouzon's syndrome to be associated with advanced paternal age.

CHARACTERISTICS

The basic defect occurring in Crouzon's syndrome is a premature fusion of the bones of the skull. Normally the bones of a baby's skull are joined together by fibrous tissue in specific places, known as 'sutures'. This comparatively loose connection of the bones of the skull allows for enlargement of the underlying brain during the early growing years and also allows for 'moulding' of the baby's head as it passes down the birth canal. In Crouzon's syndrome the early closure of these sutures results in the specific features seen in the head and faces of babies with this condition.

Head: this is small – again a fact directly due to the early closure of the bones of the skull. On feeling the baby's head, there will be no normal fontanelles – the bones of the head being of one continuous structure. (The fontanelles – two on a baby's head, anterior and posterior fontanelles – are gaps in the skull where the brain is covered only by strong fibrous tissue. These fontanelles are normally closed by around 18 months of age.) The baby's forehead is usually high and can be bulging forwards.

A **cleft palate** may also be present. In the most severe cases, underdevelopment of the external meatus of the ear can also occur.

On X-ray examination the para-nasal sinuses are also seen to be small.

Facial features: Probably the most striking facial feature of the baby with Crouzon's syndrome is the shallow orbit containing the eyes. This has the effect of causing the eyes to protrude (cf Apert's syndrome). There may also be a marked divergent squint and/or nystagmus. The optic nerve may also be damaged due to the bony abnormalities. This can result in optic atrophy with advancing blindness.

The nose is characteristically beaked and the septum dividing the two sides of the nose can be deviated to one side. This can cause obstruction to normal nasal breathing.

Teeth, when they erupt, are often overcrowded and malformed. This is due, in part, to the malformation of the jaw. The upper jaw tends to be smaller than normal. This feature, with a normal sized lower jaw tends to give the baby a pugnacious appearance.

Learning disability is regretfully a common finding in children with Crouzon's syndrome. A common complication of this condition is **increased cranial pressure** – again as a direct result of the premature closure of the bones of the skull.

The above description is of the most severely affected child. Due to the wide variation in the expressivity of the condition, less severely affected children are seen. Sometimes it is only when the skull is X-rayed that the syndrome is diagnosed.

MANAGEMENT IMPLICATIONS

In the early days of life **breathing** may be a problem if the nose is severely affected. (All new-born babies breathe solely through their noses, so any problems with this feature can have serious consequences.)

Neuro-surgical intervention will be needed, as a matter of urgency, if signs of a **raised inter-cranial pressure** occur. Signs of this will be vomiting, irritability and/or convulsions. In an older child headaches can occur or vision can become blurred. It is usual for this type of surgery to have to be undertaken during the first three months of life.

Other surgical techniques may be necessary later on in life to correct unusual facial features.

Regular **developmental checks** will need to be done to check on progress in all areas of development. In conjunction with this, regular extra checks on vision and hearing will need to be done to pick up any deterioration in these particular senses.

Schooling will need to be geared to each individual child's specific needs, taking into account the degree of mental ability, vision and hearing. Again, close liaison between education and health authorities is vital.

THE FUTURE

Life expectancy is normal for a child with Crouzon's syndrome. The quality of life will depend very much on the severity of the condition as it affects each individual.

SELF-HELP GROUPS

Cranio-facial Support Group
44 Helmsdale Road
Leamington Spa
Warwickshire CV32 7DW
(Tel. 01926 334629)

Aims and provisions: contact with other families; information and advice about this and similar conditions; practical advice and help regarding hospital visits and surgery.

'Let's Face It' (network for the facially disfigured)
10 Wood End
Crowthorne
Berkshire RG11 6DG

Aims and provisions: a junior branch of this organization links parents who have facially disfigured children.

Cystic fibrosis

ALTERNATIVE NAMES

Cystic fibrosis of pancreas; mucoviscoidosis. (Both these names are rarely used these days, but may be found in old articles.)

INCIDENCE

Cystic fibrosis is the commonest inherited condition in the UK at present. It is common in all North European populations and also in the USA. African and Asian populations rarely suffer from this condition.

The incidence in the white populations affected is as high as one live birth in every 2000 to 2500. Both boys and girls can be affected.

CAUSATION

Cystic fibrosis is inherited as an autosomal recessive. About one in 20 to one in 25 people carry the abnormal gene in the populations affected by the disease. Carriers have no symptoms of cystic fibrosis; it is only when a baby is conceived by two carriers of the condition that he/she will show the typical characteristics.

There can be several genes which show changes or mutations causing cystic fibrosis. It is thought that the degree of severity suffered is dependent upon which gene disorder is present. Active research is continuing into this, and many other, aspects of cystic fibrosis. The basic fault occurring as a result of these altered genes is in the protein CFTR. This protein is responsible for the passage of salt ions across the membranes of cells in the body. As a result of this fault, sticky mucus is produced in various organs. The lungs and pancreas are the main organs involved, but the liver and sweat glands also show changes. It is the effects of this excess of sticky mucus that gives rise to the problems seen in cystic fibrosis, together with the resultant subsequent damage to many organs in the body.

Antenatal diagnosis is possible by chorionic villus sampling and/or amniocentesis. Relatives of affected individuals can be tested for carrier status when pregnancy is being considered.

CHARACTERISTICS

One of the first signs that a baby has cystic fibrosis can be in the very early days of life. Obstruction of the bowel can occur by the build-up of sticky meconium – that waste product in the baby's bowel normally passed soon after birth. This condition is known as **meconium ileus**. Around 5% to 10% of babies with cystic fibrosis have this early complication of the disorder.

Lungs are the organs most seriously affected by cystic fibrosis. Build-up of sticky mucus in the respiratory passages, nose and sinuses as well as lungs, results in frequent and severe respiratory infections from an early age. These repeated infections will eventually cause permanent damage to the lungs. Treatment is by antibiotics for each bout of infection. But unfortunately difficult-to-treat infections, such as those caused by the *Pseudomonas* bacteria, become more common as the child matures. A vaccine against this particular form of infection is currently being evaluated.

The mainstay of treatment for the lung problems of cystic fibrosis, as well as appropriate antibiotic therapy, is regular physiotherapy on a thrice-daily basis. Through postural drainage the child is able to cough up some of the sticky mucus which is continually being accumulated in his/her lungs. Parents become very adept at giving their child this form of physio-therapy. But it can become an enormous burden to carry out this time-consuming and demanding (for both parent and child) treatment three times every day – Saturdays, Sundays, holidays and school days. In recent years, heart-lung transplants have been carried out on children with severe cystic fibrosis with a good deal of success.

In addition to the symptoms in the respiratory tract, the **digestive system** is also affected. Specific enzymes from the pancreas are deficient. This gives rise to digestive problems as food is not adequately digested and absorbed due to lack of this enzyme. So, within a few months the baby will not be thriving as well as could be expected. Weight gain is slow and anaemia due to specific malabsorption of foods containing iron can result if the diagnosis is not made and appropriate treatment given. Treatment consists of regular medication with pancreatic enzyme replacement prod-ucts. With this, and the addition of a highly nutritious diet (for which specialized dietetic advice is necessary in the early days) the child will start to gain weight. Extra salt will also need to be given, as salt is lost in excess through the sweat glands in children with cystic fibrosis. This is especially important to remember in hot weather or when the child goes abroad to a hot climate. Salt depletion can give rise to serious heat prostration.

Sweat glands in cystic fibrosis children are also involved in the generalized disorder of many glands. The excess salt that is excreted by these glands, found all over the body, is the basis for the conclusive diagnostic test for cystic fibrosis. Excess sweat, induced by a specialized technique, is analysed. Cystic fibrosis sufferers have high levels of salt loss through these glands – up to twice as high as normal.

The **liver**, the largest gland in the body and concerned very much with many aspects of metabolism, can also be affected by blockage of ducts with sticky mucus. In a few children this vital organ can become damaged by this.

Prolapse of the rectum (protrusion of part of the lower bowel at the anus) is a further clue to the diagnosis of cystic fibrosis. This occurs only in around 5% to 10% of children with cystic fibrosis, but repeated episodes of this may occur. This may be a minor problem when compared with the serious effects in the lungs and digestive system, but nevertheless a worrying one for parents. Gentle replacement of the bowel is all that is necessary.

Cystic fibrosis is a serious, life-threatening disease, but one which is being extensively researched. Hopefully, within a decade, gene therapy will be the answer to many of the problems.

MANAGEMENT IMPLICATIONS

Lung problems are the most serious aspect of cystic fibrosis. Frequent infections needing urgent and prolonged antibiotic treatment will occur. Fighting these infections, which also cause loss of appetite, will add to the problems of normal growth and weight gain. The necessary on-going physiotherapy also eats into the daily lives of both parents and children.

When school days arrive, these two aspects create difficulties. Keeping up with schoolwork, when frequent absences with respiratory infection is a fact of life, can cause problems. Sympathetic help, with suitable work sent home, and extra help at school when the child is fit, can do much to help and encourage cystic fibrosis families. Long admissions into hospital are often the lot for many cystic fibrosis children. Liaison with their local school can help to keep interest going and also prevent large sections of work being missed.

Physiotherapy in the middle of the school day can be a problem. The ways of overcoming this are many and varied, depending on local facilities. In an ideal situation, nursing or physiotherapy help can be made available for a midday physiotherapy session. At junior school, mothers can be made welcome in school to fulfil this task if the child is not able to go home for lunch. Sufficient space, of course, must also be made available in which to do the physiotherapy – often a problem for many schools. Children can learn the proper positions for their own postural drainage at a surprisingly early age. A controlled exercise programme is a vital part of the physiotherapy programme, and parents and carers should encourage the child to continue with these activities. Swimming is excellent therapy. Antibiotic treatment can be continued in school for the older cystic fibrosis child if teachers are willing to supervise medication. Older children needing intravenous antibiotic treatment can be fitted with a special device so that injections can continue whilst still attending school. Obviously the child concerned, under these circumstances, must be capable and willing to undertake this part of his/her own treatment.

Diet is also important in the management of children with cystic fibrosis. Today's thinking on this aspect of treatment is for diet to be of a high calorie nature in order to maintain growth. The help of a dietitian initially, and later in a monitoring capacity, is vital to ensure that the best combination of suitable foods are given. School meals must be monitored and teachers informed of the specific needs of their pupil with cystic fibrosis. Frequent oily, bulky, offensive stools can be a difficult problem, and may indicate that the intake of fat in the diet needs to be reduced. To help with this offensive odour at home – and at school – there are several proprietary deodorizers available commercially.

Holidays are as important for the cystic fibrosis child as anyone else, but must be geared to his/her needs. Many cystic fibrosis children pursue active sports, but these must be monitored carefully in order to avoid further damage to lung capacity. (This also applies, of course, to physical education in school.) When taking a cystic fibrosis child to a hot country, adequate salt replacement must be borne in mind.

Sexual development is often delayed in children with cystic fibrosis, often by as much as two years.

THE FUTURE

This depends very much on the severity of the disease. Many children do not survive beyond their early twenties. But with several treatment changes in view, this outlook seems set to improve within the foreseeable future.

- **Antibiotic** treatment is improving all the time;
- **Heart–lung transplants** are proving successful in prolonging life for severely affected children;
- **Gene therapy**, in which the damaged gene is replaced by a normal one,

is being actively researched and will doubtless come to fruition within the foreseeable future.

SELF-HELP GROUP

Cystic Fibrosis Research Trust
Alexandra House
5 Blythe road
Bromley
Kent BR1 3RS
(Tel. 0181 464 7211)

Aims and provisions: support and advice to families – 300 local groups; research programmes at universities and hospitals; fund raising for research; cystic fibrosis news publications; videos and films.

Down's syndrome

ALTERNATIVE NAMES

Trisomy 21; mongolism (obsolete).

INCIDENCE

Down's syndrome is the most well-known chromosomal abnormality. The overall incidence in Caucasian, Japanese and American Negro populations is between one in every 660 live births and one in every 800 live births. These are average figures, as Down's syndrome is very dependent on the age of the mother. The risk rises sharply when the age of the mother is over 35 years. Both boys and girls can be affected.

HISTORY

Down's syndrome children have been recognized for many years. In the early part of the 20th century, Dr Langdon Down specifically and accurately described all the features associated with the condition.

CAUSATION

Down's syndrome is caused by a chromosomal abnormality and there are two distinct ways in which the abnormality can arise. The commonest method occurs when an extra chromosome is added in the 21 position. Hence the name Trisomy 21. So the total chromosome count, under these conditions, will be 47 chromosomes instead of the usual 46. This occurs when chromosome pairs fail to separate during the production of the egg or sperm. This is known as 'non-dysjunction'. The risk of this occurring is greater with advancing maternal age. This effect accounts for most of the babies with Down's syndrome. But in about 5% of cases, the extra chromosome is added on to another chromosome. This is known as 'translocation'. Under these circumstances, the total chromosome count in the affected baby will be the normal 46. But there will be one 'compound' chromosome in this number. Either parent can be the carrier of a 'balanced translocation'. There is no increase in the incidence of this type of Down's syndrome baby with greater maternal age. (A balanced translocation is the situation when the individual, i.e. the mother, concerned is clinically normal.) But this compound chromosome will still exert the same clinical effects as in the baby with 47 chromosomes.

The risk of giving birth to a Down's syndrome baby, due to nondysjunction, rises with maternal age. At 30 the risk is estimated to be one in 800, whilst at 44 years this risk can be as high as one in 50. Where the syndrome is due to translocation there is no increased risk with a higher maternal age. The risk of further Down's babies is 10% when the translocation is carried by the mother and 2.5% when carried by the father.

There are other very rare forms of chromosomal disorders which can produce a Down's syndrome baby. These, of course, must be taken into account when genetic counselling is given to couples who already have a Down's syndrome child.

Antenatal diagnosis is available at around the 16th week of pregnancy by amniocentesis. Chorionic villus sampling, at ten to 12 weeks of pregnancy, is also a possible means of antenatal diagnosis. A blood test is used where there is a family history of Down's syndrome or where the mother is reaching the end of her reproductive years. Trials are under way, at specialized centres, to perfect an ultra-sound technique which can detect specific abnormalities early in pregnancy.

CHARACTERISTICS

Diagnosis of Down's syndrome can be made at birth by the very specific physical characteristics shown by these babies.

Facial features include an upward slant to the eyes with marked epicanthic folds. A small head, noticeably flatter at the back, in association with a short neck is a typical feature. Ears are small, but the tongue is large and has distinctive deep furrows on the surface.

Eye abnormalities can include cataracts, squint and nystagmus, although all these abnormalities are not always present in every child with Down's syndrome. The majority of Down's syndrome children have white flecks on the iris – Brushfield's spots. These spots cause no problems with vision, but are a helpful diagnostic feature.

Limbs are relatively short, making final height on the low side of average. Bodily proportions are normal (cf achondroplasia).

Fingers are short and stubby and have a characteristically inturning little finger in many babies. There is usually a single palmar crease. This is a common feature in children with some degree of learning disability although single palmar creases on the hands can also be found on many people with normal intellectual abilities.

Feet have a specific characteristic in that the great toe is widely separated from the other toes. This is most obvious when looking at the soles of the feet.

Muscle tone is always poor, so that Down's syndrome babies are usually 'floppy'. Subsequent physical development is slower than normal and walking occurs relatively late.

These are the specific characteristics by which a Down's syndrome baby can be recognized at birth. Confirmation will need to be done by chromosomal analysis.

As development proceeds, it becomes obvious that there is **developmental delay**. Intellectual development is often slow in the first few months or years of life, but can be within the range of normal. As the Down's syndrome child matures he/she is seen to be falling further and further behind his/her peers. Schooling can often initially take place in mainstream schools but, certainly by the time secondary school age is reached, special facilities will be found to be necessary if the child is to fulfil his/her full potential.

Personality: Most Down's syndrome children are affectionate, happy young people who are a delight to have around. They have an inherent sense of fun which can add much to family life.

Other features are frequently associated with Down's syndrome:

- **Congenital heart disease** affects around 40% of Down's syndrome babies. The most common anomalies are atrial septal defects, ventricular septal defects and/or patent ductus arteriosus.
- **Upper respiratory tract infections** are common throughout infancy and childhood. This is in part due to the smallness of the airpassages, and also due to an impaired immune system. Similarly ear infections are common and can lead to a conductive **deafness**.
- **Thyroid disease**, both hypo- and hyper-thyroidism occurs in about 20% of Down's syndrome children. The former is the most common.
- **Acute lymphatic leukaemia** has a higher incidence in Down's children, and is responsible for around 5% of deaths in early childhood.

MANAGEMENT IMPLICATIONS

Learning disability: This consistent feature of Down's syndrome children needs careful assessment and management. The infant and young child will be maturing along the same lines as his/her peers, although at a progressively slower rate. So, it is important that suitable playthings for the developmental stage reached and not the chronological age should be provided.

Physiotherapy help is important early on in the life of the child with Down's syndrome. Help can be given to encourage movement, and also to advise parents on the management of their hypotonic baby. The activities suggested will also help in the control of the recurrent respiratory tract infections to which Down's babies are particularly susceptible.

Attendance at playgroup and nursery schools can follow the usual pattern, and many Down's syndrome children manage very adequately in the lower classes of the mainstream infant school. But by the age of about seven or eight years it becomes obvious that the child is finding the work difficult. His/her small stature, poor co-ordination and relatively weak muscles all cause problems in joining in with his/her peers. It is at this time that comprehensive assessment is of great importance to determine the way forward. Some type of special schooling or extra resources will usually be found to be needed. The type of education will depend very much on what is available locally.

Down's children should live as part of a normal family if at all possible. Their affectionate, happy personality flowers within the love and security of the family unit.

Eye abnormalities: Squints need to be assessed and correction undertaken, by orthoptic or surgical means, if amblyopia is to be avoided. This is important, as Down's syndrome children need all possible sensory input to maximize their abilities.

Respiratory tract infections, which are frequently associated with middle ear infection, will need adequate and sustained treatment. Bronchitis, following on from upper respiratory tract infections, is common in Down's syndrome children, also needing adequate treatment.

Deafness, as a result of frequent middle ear disease, needs assessment and treatment. Distraction tests are usually successful in assessing hearing. Myringotomy, to remove sticky secretions from the middle ear, may be all that is necessary in the early stages. But many Down's syndrome children will need hearing aids later in life.

Thyroid disease must always be remembered when caring for a Down's syndrome child. Any excessive slowing of activity with weight gain, specific hair loss and a hoarsening of the voice, should alert carers to the possibility of hypothyroidism. Treatment with thyroxine will remedy this. Routine assessment of thyroid state throughout life is necessary to maintain correct dosage of this hormone.

Congenital heart disease will have been noted during routine medical checks. If a defect has been found, regular follow-up, and appropriate treatment if necessary, should be done.

Weight control is also important for the child with Down's syndrome. Excess weight is often gained due to the relative immobility of these children. Dietetic advice is valuable.

THE FUTURE

If the first year of life is survived, Down's syndrome children have an average life expectancy of around 40 to 50 years, although ages of over 60 have been attained. Mortality during the first year of life is usually due to congenital heart disease and/or respiratory tract infections. Malignancies, particularly leukaemia, account for deaths later in childhood.

Work in a sheltered environment or attendance at a special centre where suitable occupations are available, can be undertaken by Down's syndrome adults. Lives can be happy and fulfilled within such a caring environment.

It is believed that all men with Down's syndrome are infertile, and women have a low fertility.

In later life, features of Alzheimer's disease can unhappily make their appearance, adding to the difficulties of caring for these older people with Down's syndrome.

SELF-HELP GROUP

Down's Syndrome Association
155 Mitcham Road
London SW17 9PG
(Tel. 0181 682 4001)

Aims and provisions: to provide information, advice and counselling; to find occupations and to make people with Down's syndrome 'people with prospects'; local conferences and meetings; numerous publications.

Duchenne muscular dystrophy

ALTERNATIVE NAMES

Childhood pseudohypertrophic muscular dystrophy; progressive muscular dystrophy.

INCIDENCE

The disease affects males only; the number with this progressive condition is variable and ranges between one in every 1500 and one in every 7500. In the USA, Australia and Japan the average incidence of Duchenne muscular dystrophy is thought to be one in every 3300 live-born boys.

There are a number of other neuromuscular disorders which have similar characteristics, but Duchenne muscular dystrophy is by far the commonest type to be found in childhood.

HISTORY

The typical signs and symptoms of Duchenne muscular dystrophy were described as long ago as 1861. In 1943 the X-linked pattern of inheritance was determined; in 1983, the exact site of the gene on the X chromosome was located.

CAUSATION

Duchenne muscular dystrophy is inherited usually as an X-linked recessive condition so that only boys are affected, with about two-thirds of mothers being carriers. But new mutations can also give rise to the condition. The basic fault is the defect of a specific protein found in muscle fibres, known as 'dystrophin'. The absence of this protein in specific parts of the muscle probably allows leakage of specific enzymes, such as creatine kinase, into the bloodstream. The presence of high levels of creatine kinase in a blood sample of an affected child is confirmative proof of Duchenne muscular dystrophy.

Antenatal diagnosis can be made by first of all determining the sex of the baby. Then, if the baby is a boy, antenatal DNA studies can be done at around ten weeks of pregnancy.

Genetic counselling is of importance in families with a boy affected by Duchenne muscular dystrophy.

CHARACTERISTICS

Boys with Duchenne muscular dystrophy have no signs of the disease at birth and develop and grow normally until around 18 months of age. Between this age and three years the characteristic clinical features of the condition make their appearance.

Walking: there may be some delay in the onset of this skill – at 18 months or later. (The normal age of learning to walk is, of course, very variable, and normal times range from nine months to two years. Nevertheless, any boy who is not showing definite signs of being able to walk at 18 months should be carefully watched for further signs of Duchenne muscular dystrophy.)

By three years of age the diagnosis is usually obvious. The boy will have a waddling gait with a marked **lumbar lordosis** and will still be having frequent falls. He will have great difficulty in running (if he can at all) and will also find climbing stairs a problem. The classical sign of Duchenne muscular dystrophy occurs as the affected boy tries to get up onto his feet again after a fall. He will push his legs out behind him, and place his hands on the floor in front. He will then 'walk' his hands up to his legs to push himself into the upright position. This is known as the 'Gower manoeuvre'. These difficulties in walking and associated activities are due to weakness of the pelvic and leg muscles. The muscles of the calves of the legs of boys with Duchenne muscular dystrophy are often enlarged, giving the false appearance of power. This enlargement is due to an infiltration of the muscle by fibrous and fatty tissue. (This is the reason behind the alternative name of pseudohypertrophic muscular dystrophy.) The tendons (Achilles tendon) at the heel are tight in boys with muscular dystrophy and this adds to the walking difficulties.

Other **muscles** of the body also become progressively involved in the disease process. Muscles of the shoulders, arms and chest become weakened and movements of all kinds become more and more difficult.

Chest deformities and scoliosis can occur and breathing also eventually becomes affected due to the weakness of the intercostal muscles which are closely involved in the normal breathing process. Due to this involvement of the respiratory muscles, bronchitis and pneumonia are more likely to occur.

Heart muscle is not exempt from the generalized musculature problems, and congestive heart failure can occur due to this.

Specific learning difficulties, dyslexia in particular, can occur in a minority of boys with Duchenne muscular dystrophy. It is thought that about one-third of boys with the condition may have this added problem.

Investigations

Specific investigations are available which confirm the clinical diagnosis of Duchenne muscular dystrophy:

- **Creatine kinase** levels in the blood are very high, often up to ten times the normal level for this enzyme. These high levels are always present in the very earliest stages of the disease. Over the succeeding years the level falls but never reaches normal values.
- **ECG** abnormalities are seen in the tracing in 70% to 90% of boys with Duchenne muscular dystrophy.
- **Electromyelogram** and **muscle biopsy** of affected muscles are always found to be abnormal.

Regrettably, Duchenne muscular dystrophy is a progressive disease, and sufferers become wheelchair bound by the time they reach ten to 12 years of age. Death from respiratory infection or cardiac failure is the usual tragic outcome by the early twenties or before.

MANAGEMENT IMPLICATIONS

At present there is no cure for Duchenne muscular dystrophy. But much can be done to improve the quality of life for the boy with Duchenne muscular dystrophy.

Moderate **exercise** within the limits of possible movement is important in the early years of the disease. Exercise which is too strenuous should be avoided, however, as this will only accelerate the breakdown of muscle tissue. Immobilization of any kind will lead to the risk of joint contractures, and may also encourage obesity, which in turn will add to respiratory problems. Physiotherapy is of immense value and should be given top priority in the early stages of the condition. Passive stretching of hip, knee and ankle joints should be done and parents should be taught how to continue this on a regular basis. Similarly, good breathing habits should be taught, and boys (and their parents!) encouraged to practise these, again, on a regular daily basis.

Later, as the disease progresses inexorably, a suitable **wheelchair** will be necessary. Electrically propelled chairs will make the child more self-sufficient once he is able to manage this piece of equipment. Attention must be paid to the correct size of the wheelchair. The seating part of the chair is of particular importance in the prevention of scoliosis with all its possible attendant chest problems.

Skin care is especially important, as with the loss of muscle bulk and accompanying weight loss the skin becomes very fragile.

Home modifications for sleeping and toileting purposes may need to be considered as the child matures.

Schooling with special facilities available for wheelchairs must be organized. The boy with Duchenne muscular dystrophy will need to be encouraged to take interest in non-physical activities. The help of an **occupational therapist** is also of value for this purpose.

Chest infections and possible **heart failure** must receive urgent and on-going medical attention.

Constipation can be a minor, but irritating problem of life in a wheelchair. Diet, with perhaps a suitable occasional medication for this purpose, should be successful in eliminating this uncomfortable problem.

Support from a specialist social worker is valuable if this is possible. Financial assistance can be sorted out together with short-term residential respite care to allow other members of the family to have an active holiday.

Emotional support for the family from all involved, in whatever capacity, is a very real necessity. The progressive nature of the disease, with the very poor life expectancy, can make coming to terms with the facts extremely difficult. Both parents and the boy will need continuing sensitive support, especially if a brother has already died from the condition, or there is a further family member who is in a later stage of the disease.

THE FUTURE

A wheelchair existence from around ten to 12 years of age and an early death from cardiac or respiratory failure, is the depressing outlook for boys with Duchenne muscular dystrophy. However, a positive approach with adequate support can vastly improve the quality of life for the whole family.

SELF-HELP GROUPS

Duchenne Family Support Group
37a Highbury New Park
Islington
London N5 2EN
(Tel. 0171 704 0142)

Aims and provisions: support and advice to families; events organized for families; annual general meetings and speakers on issues relating to disease.

A further group involved in all types of muscular dystrophy is:

Muscular Dystrophy Group
Nattrass House
35 Macaulay Road
London SW4 0QP
(Tel. 0171 720 8055)

Aims and provisions: practical and emotional support through family care officers; fundraising activities; publications on various aspects of muscular dystrophy.

For help about suitable equipment, contact:

Disabled Living Foundation
346 Kensington High Street
London W14 8NS

Edward's syndrome

ALTERNATIVE NAMES

Trisomy 18.

INCIDENCE

In the USA and UK the incidence of Edward's syndrome is reported to be one in every 6600 live births. Edward's syndrome is a chromosomal abnormality which can be divided into three groups according to the severity of the condition.

- The most severe form, where the majority of cells in the body show the abnormality. The baby is severely disabled and has only a very short life expectancy.
- The 'mosaic' form, in which some cells in the body have a normal chromosome complement whilst others have the typical chromosomal pattern of the severe form of Edward's syndrome. These babies are less severely affected and have a longer life expectancy, although this does not usually extend beyond ten years of age.
- A milder, or partial, form of the condition depending on the part of the chromosome affected. These babies can show few signs of abnormality and will only have minimal disability.

Girls are marginally more often affected than boys by Edward's syndrome.

CAUSATION

Babies born with Edward's syndrome have 47 chromosomes instead of the usual complement of 46. The extra chromosome is in the 18 position (cf Down's syndrome). There seems to be an increased number of babies born with Edward's syndrome born to older mothers.

Chorionic villus sampling can diagnose the syndrome at nine to 12 weeks of pregnancy, whilst amniocentesis at 16 weeks shows the unusual chromosome count in the aspirated amniotic fluid. During the pregnancy of an Edward's syndrome baby there is frequently an excess of amniotic fluid. The baby tends to move less than a normal baby does during the latter months of pregnancy. A further unusual feature that has been noted is that pregnancies with an Edward's syndrome baby often tend to last longer than the usual 40 weeks. It is of importance that chromosomal analysis is done on the cells of an affected baby to be certain of the diagnosis. The serious implications of the finding of an extra chromosome 18 can then be faced and appropriate care and support of the family given.

CHARACTERISTICS

These can be multiple and many of the manifestations can be found in other syndromes. So it is important that all the features are considered together before a definite diagnosis is made, supported eventually by chromosomal analysis.

All babies with the severe form of trisomy 18 are **developmentally delayed** with **severe learning disability**. Other babies with the mosaic, or partial, forms may have varying degrees of learning disability or have normal intellectual abilities.

Many of the babies are **hypotonic** at birth, and this can cause **feeding difficulties** because of inability to suck adequately. Following on from this, weight gain and growth in general is slow.

After the neonatal period has passed, babies with Edward's syndrome become **hypertonic**.

As many as 95% of severely affected babies have a **congenital heart defect**, a ventricular septal defect or a patent ductus arteriosus being the two most commonly seen abnormalities.

Hands and **feet** both show very specific abnormalities. The baby with Edward's syndrome usually holds his fists tightly clenched with the fourth and fifth fingers overlapping the other fingers. There is also often a single palmar crease and the markings on the finger tips is unusual. Feet are convex on the soles and are termed 'rockerbottom' feet. Heels are also particularly prominent, adding to the unusual shape.

Renal abnormalities are also common in babies with Edward's syndrome. Horseshoe kidneys are found in over 50% of babies. Renal problems may not become apparent within the first few weeks of life or may be so severe as to cause early renal failure.

Facial features include lowset and unusually shaped ears, a short neck and small jaw. The diameter between the parietal bones of the skull is also small, and this can be a diagnostic feature on ultrasound in the antenatal period.

MANAGEMENT IMPLICATIONS

It is vital that the correct diagnosis is made by chromosomal analysis so that parents can be told of the problems that may be encountered as their baby grows. Support and sensitive counselling will be necessary for those parents who have a severely affected baby who is not expected to live more than a few months.

Feeding difficulties will need to be addressed in the early days and nasogastric feeding may be necessary initially due to the poor suck and excessive tiring of the hypotonic baby. Feeding with expressed breast-milk is preferable.

Respiratory difficulties frequently occur and will need specialized treatment in the early days of life.

Congenital heart disease, so commonly found, will need accurate diagnosis and assessment. Incipient cardiac failure must be treated and future surgery contemplated depending, of course, on the general condition of the baby.

Learning disability will need to be fully assessed at a later date, and developmental 'milestones' carefully checked in an on-going manner in the less severely affected child.

THE FUTURE

For babies with the severe form of Edward's syndrome life is short and death usually occurs within the first few weeks or months of life. With the partial form, however, the outlook is less grim. Depending on the severity of the condition the child may live into the teenage years, or even longer. Disability will again depend on the severity of the condition.

Following the birth of a baby with Edward's syndrome, genetic counselling before a further pregnancy is indicated.

SELF-HELP GROUP

SOFT UK
Froggarts Ride
Walmley
Sutton Coldfield
West Midlands B76 8TQ
(Tel. 0121 351 3122)

Aims and provisions: support, advice and information for affected families; bereavement support; encourages research; creates public awareness of Edward's syndrome.

Ehlers–Danlos syndrome

ALTERNATIVE NAME

Joint laxity.

INCIDENCE

This is a very rare syndrome, the incidence in the UK being in the region of one in every 50 000 live births. The number of cases in other parts of the world has not been accurately assessed.

There are a number of sub-types of the Ehlers–Danlos syndrome, with nine having been described to date. As research into the condition proceeds it is possible that a number of further variants will be found. However, all types have some disorder of the connective tissues of the body in common. This includes problems with skin and joints in the main, but in some types blood vessels and internal organs can also be affected. Both boys and girls can be affected equally in most variants. The exception to this is Ehlers–Danlos type 5, where only boys are affected due to the mode of inheritance.

HISTORY

International research is being carried out into this syndrome. Much initial work was done in the 1970s and 1980s.

CAUSATION

Ehlers–Danlos syndrome is a genetic condition, most types being inherited as an autosomal dominant with, at present, the exception of Ehlers–Danlos 5, which is an X-linked recessive condition.

Antenatal diagnosis is not currently available. Ehlers–Danlos syndrome is not immediately apparent at birth, but does become noticeable in early childhood.

It is probable that a specific enzyme defect is the basic cause of this syndrome.

CHARACTERISTICS

All types of Ehlers–Danlos syndrome have the following two characteristics.

Joint hypermobility: many of the joints of the body can be put through an extraordinarily wide range of movements. For example, thumbs can easily be pulled back onto the forearm. This is primarily due to the laxity of the ligaments surrounding the joints. As a result of this extreme looseness, joints are easily dislocated on minimal injury. In some types of the Ehlers–Danlos syndrome, bones become deformed due to the lack of support around the joints by capsules and ligaments. Probably the most obvious example of this is the extreme flat feet (pes planus) seen in some children, and adults, with this condition. Severe scoliosis can also be a worrying feature again due to the lack of support around the vertebral joints by ligaments.

The **skin** can be pulled away easily from the underlying tissues and is especially fragile. Hence injury is common with minimal trauma. Bruising occurs frequently, due both to skin fragility and to abnormalities in the walls of the underlying bloodvessels. Damage to skin is particularly likely to occur over bony prominences such as elbows and knees and also where skin is stretched tightly over underlying bones such as the shins and the forehead. Healing of wounds can also take longer than usual, again due to general tissue fragility. Scars are paper thin, and so are prone to recurrent injury.

Other problems encountered in different sub-types of the Ehlers–Danlos syndrome include the following:

- **Arteries**: in one type of this syndrome these important blood vessels are especially affected. The walls are thin and easily ruptured. This is a potentially dangerous situation, and can lead to fatalities.
- **Teeth** and the surrounding gums are especially affected in another type of this syndrome. Teeth become loose at an early age due to repeated gum infections. Because of this, teeth may need to be extracted at an early age.
- **Eyes** can also be affected by the generalized disorder of connective tissue. Detachment of the retina, leading to rapid loss of vision unless treated urgently, is common.

All of these effects are not necessarily to be found in any one child suffering from Ehlers–Danlos syndrome. The sub-type present determines which connective tissues are predominantly affected.

MANAGEMENT IMPLICATIONS

Joint and skeletal effects: due to the ease with which joints can dislocate, contact sports and physical activities which put excessive strain on joints should be avoided. Rapid reduction of dislocated joints, when and if they occur, is important. Scoliosis, if present, will benefit from orthopaedic advice, as will flat feet. Physiotherapy to strengthen muscles surrounding joints is important.

Skin will need similar careful treatment. Any activity where skin lacerations or bruising have a high probability of occurring should be avoided as far as is possible. This, of course, is incredibly difficult to avoid in the rough and tumble of childhood. But preventative measures such as protective padding or clothing over bony prominences, such as elbows and knees, can avoid at least some of the injury. Sympathetic handling is often needed to persuade the child with Ehlers–Danlos syndrome to wear such protective clothing. If injury to the skin does occur and needs stitching, closure of the wound with tape is the preferred method of treatment. Routine stitching can give rise to further problems with healing. If surgery for any reason has to be undertaken, particular care will be needed to ensure that adequate healing takes place.

Teeth: meticulous and on-going dental care is vital for children and adults with Ehlers–Danlos syndrome. The probable early loss of teeth with some types makes good fitting and maintenance of dentures a priority.

Eyes: retinal detachment must be suspected and excluded if there is any sudden loss of vision.

THE FUTURE

Children with Ehlers–Danlos syndrome will need to be protected from injury as far as possible without compromising their spontaneous energies. This will need the sympathetic co-operation of playmates as well as knowledge and understanding of their condition by teaching staff. Careers advice will need to be geared towards more sedentary occupations.

Pregnancy can often result in premature birth due to early rupture of the membranes which, at this time, are also involved in the general connective tissue abnormality.

Life expectancy is normal in Ehlers–Danlos syndrome with the exception of the type in which there is particular fragility of the large blood vessels. Here, rupture can lead to a fatal outcome.

SELF-HELP GROUP

Ehlers–Danlos Support Group
1 Chandler Close
Richmond
North Yorkshire DL10 5QQ
(Tel. 01748 823867)

Aims and provisions: mutual support of affected families by telephone and letter; information about condition; leaflets and tapes; list of specialists with particular interest in condition.

Ellis–Van Creveld syndrome

ALTERNATIVE NAME

Chondro-ectodermal dysplasia.

INCIDENCE

The Ellis–Van Creveld syndrome is a rare disorder which has been reported in many countries (the only exception to the rarity of the disease is to be found in an Amish group of people in Pennsylvania. Probably at least part of the reason for this is the high rate of inter-marriage). Both sexes are equally affected. Ultra-sound scanning after the 16th week of pregnancy can show the extra fingers on the hands which are a feature of the condition.

HISTORY

This condition was described by Ellis and Van Creveld in 1940.

CAUSATION

This syndrome is inherited as an autosomal recessive condition.

CHARACTERISTICS

Short stature is one of the main features of the Ellis–Van Creveld syndrome. Adult height ranges from 3 feet (90 cms) to 5 feet (150 cms) maximum.

The trunk is of normal proportions. The lack of height is caused by shortening of the arms below the elbows and the legs below the knees. These features are noticeable at birth. These measurements lead to an unbalanced appearance as the child matures (cf achondroplasia and hypochondroplasia).

As the child starts to walk, **knock-knees** will become very apparent. This, together with the short legs, makes for an unusual gait.

Extra **fingers** are a further constant feature of the condition. The extra fingers are usually well-developed. This is somewhat unusual, as extra digits, when found, are frequently little more than tags of skin. In a small percentage of babies (about 10%) extra **toes** are also present.

Fingernails and **toenails** are small and under-developed, and remain so throughout life.

Teeth erupt early, are of an unusual rounded barrel shape and are widely spaced. (Some babies are born with teeth already erupted. This can lead to difficulties at times with breast feeding).

Over half the babies born with this syndrome have also a congenital **heart defect**. This most frequently takes the form of an atrial septal defect – that is, an opening between the two upper chambers of the heart. This can lead to heart failure within the first few months of life, which can be fatal. About one-third of babies born with the Ellis–Van Creveld syndrome die within the first few months of life due to this cause.

MANAGEMENT IMPLICATIONS

The **short stature**, particularly if the final height is no more than 3 feet, can cause problems both at school and in later life. Chairs and tables at school will need to be adjusted to suit the child's lack of height once reception class days are over.

Sensitive handling when sports and other physical activities are undertaken is necessary. Very short children can become very frustrated by their inability to keep up with all the activities that their peers seem to so enjoy. Encouragement should be given both by parents and teachers, to try to find suitable and enjoyable hobbies for the child with the Ellis–Van Creveld syndrome. Later in life, stairs, ticket machines and cupboards – to mention just a few – will all cause problems for the adult with short stature.

Extra fingers (and toes, if present) will need to be surgically removed at some time during the early years and certainly before school days arrive.

Surgery on the congenital **heart** defect will be necessary as soon as the baby is fit enough to withstand this procedure.

If the **knock-knees** are very marked and causing difficulty in walking, orthopaedic advice will be necessary with possible operative procedures. Physiotherapy following operation will be valuable in strengthening weak muscles and to encourage good posture and walking patterns.

Genetic counselling before further pregnancies is advisable.

THE FUTURE

If there are no cardiac lesions or if these have been dealt with successfully, life expectancy is good. Careers where short stature is not a problem need to be looked into as adulthood approaches.

SELF-HELP GROUP

Ellis–Van Creveld Foundation
Farthingale Farm
Hackmans Lane
Purleigh
Essex CM3 6RW
(Tel. 01621 828914)

Aims and provisions: support and advice for families; information on the condition; data compilation on the condition to facilitate research; newsletter.

Epidermolysis bullosa

ALTERNATIVE NAMES

There are a number of sub-types of this condition, for example epidermolysis bullosa Mendes da Costa and epidermolysis bullosa Koebner type, but all have the prefix 'epidermolysis bullosa' or EBS.

INCIDENCE

The true incidence of epidermolysis bullosa is not entirely clear. In the USA a specific number of large families have been documented, many of whom have the condition. From these studies it is estimated that there are at least 50 000 Americans, mainly children, suffering from epidermolysis bullosa. It is thought that there are around 2500 sufferers in the UK.

CAUSATION

EBS is inherited as an autosomal dominant except for the two sub-types – EBS lethal type (causing early infant death), which is inherited in an autosomal manner and EBS Mendes da Costa, which is an X-linked recessive condition. The latter thus affects boys only, but boys and girls can be equally affected otherwise.

At present there is no antenatal diagnosis available apart from sampling the baby's skin at around 18 weeks of pregnancy. Genetic counselling is advisable if there is a family history of the condition.

CHARACTERISTICS

This condition affects only the **skin** and can clinically be divided into a 'simple' type and a 'dystrophic' type, depending on which layer of the skin is involved. Both types result in blistering from minimal injury.

In the **simple** type there is a wide variation in the degree of injury which produces blistering. Some babies may arrive in the world with a blistered skin due to the trauma of delivery. In others it is not until the crawling stage that any problems are encountered. In the latter circumstance the movements of clothing, on knees and elbows in particular, when crawling is sufficient to cause blistering. Scarring does not occur in this type.

In the **dystrophic** type the degree of trauma again varies very much from individual to individual. Scarring is the usual outcome after healing in this type of EBS and can be severe, giving rise to contractures and maybe loss of finger and toenails.

Depending on the sub-type, the blistering may occur anywhere on the body or be confined to the extremities.

The **mucous membrane** in the mouth may be involved in the young baby, but fortunately this does usually improve in later childhood. Soft, mashed foods should be given for as long as is necessary depending on the severity of the condition in the mouth.

Problems can arise when blisters become infected, and this can occur all too readily during the active 'into-everything' toddler years.

Other abnormalities can include **erosions and narrowing of the oesophagus**, which can give rise to difficulties with swallowing and **contractures in the joints**, which can also occur in some children with epidermolysis bullosa. This can cause a degree of disability later in life.

MANAGEMENT IMPLICATIONS

The mainstay of coping with a child with EBS is the avoidance of injury as far as possible. The unavoidable bumps and falls of childhood cause greater problems than normal. Treatment of resultant blistering must be treated with great care to avoid infection. Children's skin differs from that of adults, in that resistance to certain bacteria is weaker and so infection is a greater hazard. With increasing maturity, the blistering tends to improve and the susceptibility to infection diminishes.

School teachers should be alerted to the dangers to which their EBS pupils are exposed following even minor injury. Professional advice is a wise move if injury does occur at school. Teachers should remember that the usual sticking plaster for minor wounds should never be used on a child with EBS. On removal of the protective dressing, the abnormal skin will be painfully damaged.

An **adequate intake of food** must be maintained for the child with severe EBS. It is all too easy for nutritional deficiencies to arise due to eating problems in the early years. Children do not take readily to eating an adequate diet when their mouths are sore and eating is painful.

Some sports with much physical contact are unsuitable for children with EBS. Other activities, such as swimming, dancing and routine exercises are better for, and enjoyed by, these children.

Many facets of everyday life can be affected by EBS, for example ironing can present a problem to the sufferer of the disease, as the pressure needed to be exerted on the iron is sufficient in many cases to cause blistering with all its potential problems. Antibiotic creams will help reduce the possible dangers of infection in a blistered lesion to a minimum.

Teeth-cleaning can also cause blistering and soreness of the gums. A soft toothbrush should be used. Good dental care is vital and teeth should be preserved in the mouth at all costs. It is not possible for a sufferer from EBS to wear dentures.

Itching can sometimes be a feature of EBS, especially if the child becomes too hot. Avoidance of overheating is important under these conditions, with perhaps an anti-histamine to reduce the irritation.

THE FUTURE

EBS does tend to improve with maturity. As they grow older, sufferers will also learn how to avoid the injuries which they have found are likely to cause blistering.

Career prospects will be limited depending on the severity of the disease. For example, repetitive work needing the continual handling of objects will need to be avoided. Sheltered workshops or suitable work from home should be investigated for the EBS school-leaver.

Life expectancy is not diminished by EBS (except for the lethal form when death occurs in infancy).

SELF-HELP GROUP

DEBRA
13 Wellington Business Park
Crowthorne
Berkshire RG11 6LS
(Tel. 01344 771961)

Aims and provisions: support and advice for sufferers and their families.

Fabry disease

ALTERNATIVE NAMES

Fabry-Anderson disease; angiokeratoma; alphagalactosidase A deficiency.

INCIDENCE

Due to the complicated inheritance pattern, the exact incidence of Fabry disease is unknown, but is thought to be about one in every 40 000 live births. All races have reported the condition amongst their populations, with the exception of the American Indians. The disease usually only affects boys; reports of symptoms in carrier girls are very rare.

CAUSATION

Fabry disease is a metabolic condition in which there is a defective activity of a specific enzyme concerned with the metabolism of certain lipids in the body. As a result of this there is excessive deposition of these specific lipids in the walls of the blood vessels and also in other parts of the body. This in turn gives rise to the symptoms seen in this disease.

Inheritance of Fabry disease is as an X-linked recessive condition. There is a wide variety in the severity of the symptoms in each individual. Carrier girls can be affected but this is rare; again symptoms may range from completely absent to severe.

The condition can be diagnosed antenatally by chorionic villus sampling, or amniocentesis.

CHARACTERISTICS

The first signs of Fabry disease are usually seen in childhood. The child will complain of **pain** felt first in fingers and toes and then extending up the arms and legs, and maybe also across the abdomen and in the genital region. The pain is described as tingling or burning in character and can be very severe. The length of time for which these very unpleasant symptoms last also varies from minutes to weeks. There may be a low-grade fever associated with each episode of pain. These painful events are often triggered off by excessive tiredness, an intercurrent infection or even by a rapid change in environmental temperature, such as coming into a hot room from a cold temperature outside. Children with these symptoms will often ask to go outside in the cold again. These periodic attacks of pain tend to become less frequent during adolescence and adult life. Many people with Fabry disease will complain of permanent discomfort in hands and feet. This is often said to be worse in the late afternoon and evening.

Skin: at around the same time as these unpleasant sensations occur, clusters of dark red spots make their appearance – angiokeratomas. They can occur anywhere on the body, but most typically are seen in the greatest number in the lower part of the trunk and upper part of the legs.

Eyes: in later childhood, opaque areas, arising in whorls, are seen to be present in the cornea on examination under a slitlamp. These will cause a degree of blurred vision depending on their severity. As well as these opacities, dilated and tortuous blood vessels can be seen coursing over the conjunctiva. On ophthalmoscopic examination, similarly damaged blood vessels can be seen in the retina.

Renal complications due to the involvement of the blood vessels of the kidney can occur in late childhood and early adult life. There is gradual deterioration of kidney function and renal failure can occur at any time from the 10th birthday onwards.

Heart: the coronary blood vessels are also involved in the generalized abnormality due to the enzyme defect. This can result in coronary heart disease. Valvular heart disease – most frequently a prolapse of the mitral valve – is also associated more frequently with Fabry disease. In a similar way, **strokes** can occur from damaged cerebral blood vessels.

Other more unusual symptoms can include:

- nausea and vomiting, diarrhoea and abdominal pain due to depositions of abnormal lipids in the abdominal tissues;
- Perthes disease due to avascular necrosis of the head of the femur;
- delay in normal growth and in puberty in badly affected boys;
- excessive fatigue and weakness throughout childhood in those severely affected;
- chronic airway obstruction in severely affected children, due to the

accumulation of specific substances in the lining of the airways, causing breathing difficulties.

The symptoms and signs of Fabry disease can be wide-ranging and severe leading to a good deal of difficulty in diagnosis. A firm diagnosis can be made by finding very high levels of the specific substances which are being incompletely metabolized in the blood.

MANAGEMENT IMPLICATIONS

The **painful episodes** in limbs and other parts of the body can be relieved by giving certain specific drugs – carbamazepine, for example. Other ways of helping children through these unpleasant symptoms is to be sure that they do not become too hot and to try to avoid sudden changes in temperature as far as possible. Again, making sure that they do not get over-tired will help reduce the number of incidents of pain.

Children and parents can also be reassured that as they get older these episodes will become less frequent.

The **renal** and **heart** complications which can occur in later childhood need to be treated appropriately as they occur. Renal dialysis and kidney transplantation may be necessary in later life.

THE FUTURE

Until kidney transplantation became available, death usually occurred in the forties due to renal failure. Life expectancy can now be improved unless the heart is severely affected or a stroke is suffered.

Within the limits of disability, most careers can be followed, except those in which extreme ranges of temperature are found.

Enzyme replacement therapy is being researched and in the future will perhaps lead to a 'cure' for Fabry disease.

SELF-HELP GROUP

There is no specific self-help group, but the following group will give advice and help:

Research Trust for Metabolic Disease in Children (RTMDC)
Golden Gates Lodge
Weston Road
Crewe
Cheshire CW1 1XN
(Tel. 01270 250221)

Foetal alcohol syndrome

INCIDENCE

Amazingly, this syndrome is said to affect to some degree one in every 100 babies born in Western countries. This incidence can vary from place to place depending on the drinking habits of the local population. If the drinking habits of the mother during pregnancy are very heavy, as many as one in three babies will be affected to some extent.

HISTORY

The specific characteristics shown by babies born to mothers who drink heavily during pregnancy have only been fairly recently described in detail. The amount of alcohol needed to be consumed before demonstrable effects are seen in the baby are not clearly determined. The result will also depend on both the mother's and the baby's susceptibility to the effects of alcohol.

CAUSATION

Alcohol, and its derivatives, can cross the placenta and so exert damaging effects on the developing child. The unborn baby does not have the necessary enzymes to 'detoxify' these substances readily and will be susceptible to the adverse effects long after the alcohol has been eliminated from the mother's system. In addition to this direct effect, there can be other indirect problems. Malnutrition, dehydration and a poorly functioning placenta, all due to excess alcohol intake, can all add to the adverse effects.

The developmental problems arise early in pregnancy, when maximum laying down of vital organs occurs even before the mother herself is aware that she is pregnant. The severity of the problem will depend on both the timing during the pregnancy and the amount of alcohol taken. So it is important that drinking habits are controlled in all women who may expect to become pregnant in the foreseeable future. Defects due to this cause are probably one of the most obviously preventable of learning disability.

CHARACTERISTICS

Small size: babies who are born to heavy drinking mothers are often 'light for dates', i.e. they weigh less than would be expected for the length of pregnancy. Also they are frequently born prematurely. These babies are also slow to grow during the early months, not 'catching up' on weight and length as do most babies who are born before time.

Facial features are quite specific for babies born with the foetal alcohol syndrome. The forehead is narrow, often with small eyes and drooping eyelids which give a sleepy appearance. The top lip is long and smooth, without the 'rosebud' appearance common in babies. The lower jaw can be small.

Learning disability frequently, but not invariably, occurs.

Many babies are **irritable** during the early weeks. Later they can become **hyperactive** and easily distractible. **Speech delay** has also been reported.

There is a wide range of these effects, but all children exposed to excess levels of alcohol before birth will show developmental delay and will probably not reach their full genetic potential.

Hearing may be affected, as there is sometimes specific malfunction of the Eustachian tube, that tiny tube linking the back of the throat with the middle ear.

Other possible effects are that babies have been noted to be very **hairy** at birth; **squints** are common; and increased susceptibility to **infections** of all kinds has been noted.

MANAGEMENT IMPLICATIONS

Small size: children with the foetal alcohol syndrome will grow along the lower centiles of the growth charts and there is little that can be done to accelerate growth. This persists throughout childhood.

Learning disability: close watch must be kept on all aspects of development. Lagging behind in some aspects of the normal developmental process can be the first clue to diagnosis and so to subsequent development. Fuller assessment of areas of detected delay should be undertaken and appropriate help given to ensure that the child's full potential is reached. Speech therapy is frequently needed for speech delay.

Infections of all kinds, but most usually those connected with the respiratory tract, need to be swiftly and adequately treated whenever they occur.

Hearing must be checked routinely and continued to be monitored on a regular basis, due to the potential Eustachian tube problems. This is especially necessary following a cold.

General care and nutrition of babies born to mothers with a drink problem must always be at the forefront of the health professionals' minds throughout childhood. The mother may need help both to overcome her drinking problem and also to care adequately for her child. Health and social workers should co-operate fully to ensure that the child's safety, health and development are not adversely affected by a possible continuing drink problem.

THE FUTURE

This is very much dependent upon the care received during infancy and childhood as well as the severity, or otherwise, of the alcohol effects. Also, unless parents can be persuaded to give up their excessive drinking habits, the child, by imitation, can easily grow up into a similar pattern. Much education needs to be done on the adverse effects of heavy drinking during pregnancy.

SELF-HELP GROUPS

There are no specific group for mothers during pregnancy, but the following offer support and advice for people with drink problems:

Alcoholics Anonymous
PO Box 1
Stonebow House
Stonebow
York Y01 2NJ
(Tel. 01904 644026)

Al-Anon/Alateen Family Group
61 Dover Street
London SE1 4YT
(Tel. 0171 403 0888)

Aims: self-help for families and friends of those with a drink problem.

Fragile X syndrome

ALTERNATIVE NAMES

Martin-Bell X-linked mental retardation; fragile X chromosome.

INCIDENCE

It is thought that learning disability due to the fragile X syndrome occurs in approximately one in every 2000 to 3000 male births. This is a very high figure, so this cause of learning disability in boys is thought to be one of the most common. Girls are also affected, but to a lesser degree due to the mode of inheritance. Only 30% to 40% of girls carrying this genetic abnormality will have some degree of learning disability.

HISTORY

In 1943 Martin and Bell first published accounts of a sex-linked form of learning disability. In the late 1960s Lubs first described a family with the characteristics now known to be associated with the fragile X syndrome. The genetics of this abnormality have subsequently been demonstrated. Previously boys with learning disability associated with few other physical features were termed as having 'pure' learning disability.

There are a number of other syndromes of a similar type linked in some way to the X chromosome. Clinical features vary in these other syndromes, but learning disability of some degree is a constant finding.

CAUSATION

The cause of the fragile X syndrome is a defect in a particular part of the X chromosome (one of the sex chromosomes). This 'fragile' site is where the gene responsible for the disorder is situated. The actual genetic transmission is complicated and has not, as yet, been clearly resolved. Many families having a child with the fragile X syndrome show a definite X-linked pattern of inheritance, i.e. the condition being passed on from a carrier mother to an affected son. But many sporadic cases are now being recognized, but they may be variations of other X-linked syndromes.

At present there is no reliable antenatal test, although chorionic villus sampling at ten weeks of pregnancy can detect the fragile X syndrome in affected boys.

CHARACTERISTICS

Learning disability: the degree of this characteristic varies markedly from child to child. In some children the disability is severe, whilst in others intelligence is on the borderline of normal. For example, there may be only mild difficulties with reading or mathematical concepts. But on the other hand, some boys can be so severely affected that characteristics such as hyperactivity, repetitive behaviour, autistic features, handflapping and speech difficulties occur. Girls with the fragile X syndrome as confirmed by chromosome studies usually have normal intelligence, although a few may be mildly disabled.

Testes in 90% of boys with the fragile X syndrome become larger than normal at puberty. This may affect one testis only. There does not appear to be any loss of normal function, although few affected men have been known to father children.

Facial features: a long, thin face is frequently associated with the fragile X syndrome in both boys and girls. Boys also tend to have large ears and a prominent forehead.

Other features can occur which aid diagnosis.

Speech is frequently specifically delayed during the early years. This can also be part of the general developmental delay seen as the child matures.

Fingers which are easily hyperextended, due to the loose connective tissue around the joints, are also often a feature of children with the fragile X syndrome.

Skin is often fine and thin.

MANAGEMENT IMPLICATIONS

All babies benefit from physical and verbal stimulation during the early growing years. This is particularly important for those children with **potential developmental delay**. Babies should be talked to from birth onwards, even though no obvious response is forthcoming. Similarly, simple games which encourage co-ordination of hands and limbs will help children develop to their full potential. Help in these areas is of particular importance to children with the fragile X syndrome.

Help from clinical psychologists can be of value in the early years if autistic or hyperactive behaviour is a problem.

Comprehensive multidisciplinary assessment, on an on-going basis, is vital to determine the areas of development in which the child is lagging behind. Where problems are detected, appropriate help can then be given in the areas of delay.

Boys will probably need special schooling facilities, although this is not always the case, some boys managing mainstream schooling quite adequately or, on occasions, with added help being available. Again, full multidisciplinary assessment is necessary to determine the most appropriate placement.

Genetic counselling for families who have a member with a proven fragile X syndrome is important.

THE FUTURE

Career and job prospects will be limited in those boys showing the most severe learning disability. Sheltered employment in a caring community or with full support from a loving home is the best option under these circumstances. For the less severely affected boys, and certainly for girls with this genetic abnormality, a wide variety of work is possible.

There is no limitation of life expectancy for children with the fragile X syndrome.

SELF-HELP GROUP

Fragile X Society
53 Winchelsea Lane
Hastings
East Sussex TN35 4LG
(Tel. 01424 813147)

Aims and provisions: support and linking of families; information and advice; promotion of research.

Friedrich's ataxia

ALTERNATIVE NAMES

Friedrich's disease; hereditary spinal ataxia; recessive spino-cerebellar degeneration.

INCIDENCE

There are a number of conditions having ataxia as the prime characteristic. Friedrich's ataxia is thought to be the most common of the hereditary ataxias. Approximately one in every 50 000 babies born are likely to be affected. Boys and girls can be affected equally.

HISTORY

The most recent work on the basic cause of Friedrich's ataxia has been done by Harding. Suggestions have been made that the disease may be a metabolic one. This differs greatly from Friedrich's original thoughts on the matter, which were that the disease was due to alcoholic excess!

Active research into Friedrich's ataxia is currently being undertaken and much work needs to be done to differentiate this form of ataxia from other conditions with somewhat similar symptoms.

CAUSATION

Friedrich's ataxia is inherited as an autosomal recessive characteristic. The gene affected is situated on chromosome 9. The pathology is one of atrophy of specific parts of the spinal cord.

Antenatal diagnosis can be made by chorionic villus sampling at eight to 12 weeks of pregnancy. Genetic counselling is advisable for families who have a member with Friedrich's ataxia.

CHARACTERISTICS

Ataxia is the most obvious characteristic of this condition. At birth and up to around the age of three years there are no signs at all of any problem. In fact, the age at which the disease first manifests itself is very variable and in some children, symptoms only develop at puberty. The unsteadiness develops first in the legs and ascends relentlessly up the body until all four limbs are affected. Accompanying this unsteadiness is weakness and an inability for the child to determine the position of his/her limbs in space, adding to the ataxic problems. Sensations of touch are also diminished, but both pain and temperature change can be felt normally. Reflexes in the legs are lost early and the plantar response is extensor. Regrettably, most Friedrich's ataxia sufferers will be wheelchair bound by the age of 25.

Eyes: nystagmus or other disturbances of eye movements are noticeable in about half the children with Friedrich's ataxia. Optic atrophy also can occur in a minority.

Deafness, although less commonly seen than other abnormalities, can add to the problems of Friedrich's ataxia sufferers.

Scoliosis and **pes planus** (flat feet) develop within a few years of the disease becoming obvious. These effects arise gradually over the years as the ataxic gait becomes more apparent.

Heart: the heart is always eventually affected in Friedrich's ataxia. This vital organ becomes hypertrophied (enlarged), and so functions less well. Breathlessness and palpitations are the symptoms most usually felt by the young person. ECG changes become obvious – left ventricular hypertrophy and T wave inversion – as the condition progresses.

Diabetes develops in a significant proportion (20%) of people with Friedrich's ataxia, at a later stage of the disease. The development of this metabolic condition is more likely to occur in children and young adults, in whom visual and hearing problems are in evidence.

MANAGEMENT IMPLICATIONS

Ataxia: the child with problems of unsteadiness when walking will need to be protected against injury from falls during the early stage of the disease. Progressive weakness of the muscles will make many physical activities difficult or impossible. Depending on the severity and rate of progression of the condition, a wheelchair will eventually become a necessity.

Physiotherapy is valuable, both to reduce skeletal deformities as far as possible and to keep weakened muscles on the move. Many sufferers have commented that bed-rest seems to make their condition worse, so confinement to bed during any bout of intercurrent infection should be reduced to a minimum.

Speech therapy can be useful in helping boys and girls to find the best way to use the muscles of articulation affected by the disease.

Vision and **hearing** must be monitored on a continuing basis. Any associated refractory defect or conductive deafness, due to infection for example, should be treated early and adequately.

Heart: cardiac function needs to be accurately diagnosed clinically and by ECG and maybe also by echocardiography. Digoxin and/or betablocker drugs are often helpful in maintaining adequate cardiac function.

Diabetes: the chances of this metabolic condition being strongly associated with Friedrich's ataxia must be remembered. Symptoms of thirst, frequent passing of urine and loss of weight must be urgently investigated and appropriate treatment given if blood-sugar levels are found to be high.

Skeletal problems of scoliosis may be so severe as to need surgery. The deformed chest, due to the spinal 'twist', can give rise to problems with respiration.

THE FUTURE

Friedrich's ataxia unfortunately pursues a relentless course with few, if any, periods of remission. Few sufferers remain out of a wheelchair by the time the early twenties are reached. A fatal outcome usually occurs before the age of 40, most frequently from cardiac complications or an intercurrent respiratory infection. But these events can vary and life expectancy is enhanced for those people with less severe symptoms, and especially those with only mild cardiac symptoms and without diabetes. Improvements in treatment of cardiac and diabetic problems have, over recent years, also resulted in greater longevity.

Career choices are limited by the degree of ataxia, both affecting large muscle groups and the muscles of articulation.

SELF-HELP GROUP

Friedrich's Ataxia Group
'Copse Edge'
Thursley Road
Elstead
Godalming
Surrey GU8 6DJ
(Tel. 01252 702864)

Aims and provisions: support and advice, together with fundraising activities; leaflets.

Galactosaemia

INCIDENCE

About one baby in every 50 000 born in the UK, the USA and Germany is affected by this metabolic disease. Ireland and Austria appear to have more babies born with this condition, whilst Japanese babies are affected very rarely. Both boys and girls can show the characteristics of galactosaemia.

CAUSATION

Galactosaemia is inherited as an autosomal recessive condition. Chromosome 9 appears to be the chromosome on which the affected gene is located. Chorionic villus sampling at nine to 12 weeks of pregnancy, followed if necessary by amniocentesis a month later, will show deficiency of the enzyme involved in this condition. It is the absence, or deficient production, of this enzyme that gives rise to the characteristic features. Galactose, a substance found in milk and milk products, is the substance which is incompletely broken down. As a result, accumulations of this and other allied substances are found in various parts of the body in children suffering from this condition.

At birth the enzyme involved in the breakdown and proper metabolism of galactose is found to be absent when a sample of blood is taken from the baby. In the USA, all babies are routinely screened for galactosaemia by this method.

CHARACTERISTICS

At birth the baby is entirely well. It is not until milk feeds are given on the second or third day of life that symptoms begin to appear.

Between four and ten days of age, the baby will become **jaundiced**, and begin to refuse his/her feeds. **Vomiting** will soon become a problem. As a result there will be a loss of weight, and the baby will become lethargic and drowsy.

One of the gravest dangers at this young age is that of overwhelming infection in any part of the body. Infections, particularly with *E. coli*, are particularly liable to afflict babies with galactosaemia. He/she will be gravely ill, and death is an ever-present threat under these conditions. Even if recovery does ensue from an infection, the baby's mental and physical development can be retarded unless the true cause of the problems are diagnosed and treated.

Cataracts can also develop in the eyes if treatment is delayed for too long.

Later problems can include **specific speech defects** and later **ovarian failure**.

Convulsions can also occur.

Treatment is by exclusion of all milk and milk products from the diet. If this is done early, within the first week or two of life, damage to the liver, brain and eyes can be avoided. If the diagnosis has been delayed and milk feeds have been given for some weeks, jaundice, vomiting and loss of weight will become a grave problem. But once milk has been removed from the diet these symptoms will improve. Regrettably, however, the cataract formation, learning disability and possible liver damage can be permanent.

Avoidance of all milk products must be maintained throughout life. There are a number of commercial replacements available, such as soya-bean products and casein hydrolysates, which will satisfy the nutritional requirements of the baby. Normal physical growth can be readily maintained on these products.

MANAGEMENT IMPLICATIONS

Early and adequate treatment of **infection** in the early days of life is of vital importance if the child is to survive. Special intensive care facilities may be needed for the babies that are very sick.

The **dietary aspect** of galactosaemia is the main problem to be faced once the baby has survived the first few traumatic weeks of life. Dietetic advice on suitable foods with which to replace galactose in the diet is a necessity for parents and child carers. As the child matures it is somewhat easier from some points of view to avoid milk products. But the child may be under pressure from peers to try and eat or drink what they are eating or drinking. It must be explained carefully to the child, and to his/her immediate friends, that this course of action will cause him/her harm.

Speech defects do seem to be more commonly found in children with galactosaemia than in the general childhood population. The help of a speech therapist is necessary under these circumstances in order that understandable speech is learned.

Any possibility of **learning disability** must be carefully assessed. Routine developmental tests should pick up any delay in any of the parameters tested. In this context, the speech delay common in this condition must be remembered. Early help with various skills in which the child has been found to be behind will be valuable. Teachers specializing in assisting pre-school children can be especially helpful. When school age comes around, assessment as to the type of school most suited to the child's abilities will need to be determined. Special schooling or a unit with special resources may be necessary for some children with galactosaemia.

When reproductive age is reached, there may be **fertility** problems. Female galactosaemia sufferers not infrequently have ovarian failure which renders them infertile. If pregnancy is achieved, genetic counselling and appropriate testing during the pregnancy are advisable.

Convulsions are not usual but, if present, will need to be treated with the appropriate anti-convulsant. Regular monitoring of any such drug regime must also be undertaken.

THE FUTURE

Provided the exclusion of milk and milk products from the diet is begun early in the new-born period, and continued throughout life, there will be few problems – apart from, of course, the nuisance value of dietary restrictions.

Communication problems can persist into adult life in spite of appropriate therapy. So when career choices have to be made, it is wise to avoid any career relying heavily on verbal communication. Infertility may also cause heartache.

SELF-HELP GROUPS

Galactosaemia Parent Support Group
31 Cotysmore Road
Sutton Coldfield
West Midlands B75 6BJ
(Tel. 0121 378 5143)

Aims and provisions: contact with other families; information and advice about the condition.

The Research Trust into Metabolic Diseases in Children (RTMDC)
Golden Gates Lodge
Weston Road
Crewe
Cheshire CW1 1XN
(Tel. 01270 250221)

This group can also give advice and help.

Gaucher disease

ALTERNATIVE NAMES

Cerebroside lipidosis; familial splenic anaemia.

INCIDENCE

There are three main types of Gaucher's disease, but type 1 is by far the most common, accounting for 90% of all cases. This will be the type discussed. (Types 2 and 3 have central nervous system and pulmonary involvement as major features. Life expectancy beyond early life is poor in these types.)

Gaucher's disease is one of the 'storage' diseases. In these diseases, certain specific substances are stored to excess in the body, and it is this that accounts for the signs and symptoms of each specific condition. In all cases of storage disease it is lack of the specific enzymes which normally break these substances down that is the basic fault causing the problems. Gaucher's disease is one of a large group of lyosomal storage disorders.

Gaucher's disease is not common – figures of one in 100 000 people have been quoted, but in Ashkenazi Jews the incidence is reported as being as high as one in 600. Also, the carrier rate in this particular group of people is thought to be as high as one in 25. Girls and boys are equally affected.

Chorionic villus sampling and/or amniocentesis can detect this disease antenatally.

CAUSATION

Gaucher's disease is inherited as an autosomal recessive characteristic. The gene concerned has been mapped to chromosome 1. The basic fault is a deficiency of the enzyme glucocerebrosidease.

CHARACTERISTICS

The typical features of Gaucher's disease can occur at any time during childhood or early adult life, although signs and symptoms can occur as early as one year of age.

An **enlarged abdomen** due to an increase in size of both liver and spleen is often the first obvious sign, and is due to the storage of the excess of unmetabolized lyosomal substances. At times the liver enlargement can give rise to **abdominal pain**. As the spleen – the organ situated high in the abdomen under the left lower ribs and concerned with the proper function of blood cells – enlarges, haematological effects occur. **Anaemia** can result due to a diminution in the red cells available to perform their oxygen carrying function. General feelings of malaise and fatigue follow when anaemia becomes severe.

Small haemorrhages into the skin and easy **bruising** can also occur due to faulty clotting mechanisms. **Nose bleeds** can also become a problem.

Bone pain and **fractures** of bones can also occur as the disease progresses. This is due to infiltration of the lyosomal substances which in turn are due to the basic enzyme deficiency.

MANAGEMENT IMPLICATIONS

As the course of this condition is so variable, not every child will require the treatment outlined. Routine medical checks and parental concern will identify needs as they arise.

Splenectomy – removal of the spleen, either completely or partially – may become necessary if anaemia and/or haemorrhages become too much of a problem. This, of course, must only be undertaken with the full co-operation of paediatrician, surgeon and haemotological department.

Any **fractures** must be treated quickly and adequately. Orthopaedic advice may also be necessary for deformities which can result from the effects on the bone of the lyosomal deposits. (In cases of suspected child abuse, the pathological nature of fractures must always be remembered in a child with Gaucher's disease.) **Bone pain** will usually settle if the affected limb is immobilized for a short period of time.

Schooling can be in mainstream school, but teachers should be aware of their pupil's inherited condition. Contact sports must be avoided, due to both the increased likelihood of fractures and also due to the possibility – albeit remote – of rupture of the enlarged spleen.

Enzyme replacement and **bone-marrow transplantation** are options which are currently being explored.

THE FUTURE

Life expectancy is not usually reduced for people with the type of Gaucher's disease described here. Genetic counselling is indicated before pregnancy is contemplated. Fractures of the neck of the femur are more likely to occur in older people with this condition. Hip replacement may be necessary in early adult life due to this complication of Gaucher's disease.

SELF-HELP GROUP

Gaucher's Association
25 West Cottages
London NW6 1RJ
(Tel. 0171 433 1121)

Aims and provisions: information on condition; support and contact between families; newsletter and annual conference.

Gilles de la Tourette syndrome

ALTERNATIVE NAMES

Tourette syndrome; multiple motor and vocal tics; coprolalia generalized tic.

INCIDENCE

It is thought that this distressing condition may be much under-diagnosed due to a variety of factors such as the varying severity of the disease, time of onset and social disability caused. Research has put the occurrence of the condition as high as between one in 2000 and one in 3000 for boys and between one in 5000 and one in 10 000 for girls. Boys would appear to be around three times as likely to be affected as girls.

CAUSATION

Gilles de la Tourette syndrome is thought to be inherited as an autosomal dominant condition, but a high proportion of sufferers have no family history, so other factors may be involved. Birth injury, or the possibility of several genes being involved, are other suggestions as to aetiology.

There are no known means of diagnosing Gilles de la Tourette syndrome other than by clinical findings.

CHARACTERISTICS

The age of onset of symptoms varies greatly, and can range from two to 21 years. The most frequent age at which problems become obvious is around seven years of age.

Tics: these are of two types:

- Motor tics – involuntary movements of face, limbs and body. These unusual movements involve eye-blinking, facial grimacing, shrugging of shoulders and head and arm jerks. For a diagnosis of Gilles de la Tourette syndrome to be made these, and other, tics must be continuously present for over a year. Many children go through a stage where one or two tics occur, maybe copied from a friend or even an elderly neighbour! But these are eventually forgotten and are not replaced by other involuntary movements.
- Vocal tics – coughing, sneezing, sucking, throat-clearing, sniffing and other unusual noises. At times the involuntary shouting of inappropriate words or phrases, including obscenities, can make life extremely difficult for parents and companions of the affected child. These obscene words and phrases (including at times obscene gestures) occur in around one-third of all children and/or adults affected by this syndrome. This is a particularly socially disabling facet of the condition, and one which cannot be readily controlled. Vocal tics generally make their appearance some time after the motor tics have become established.

Obsessive behaviour is also a common feature of this syndrome. Repetitive actions and patterns of behaviour can be a further seriously disabling problem.

Reduced attention span can also make life difficult from a teaching point of view.

The whole pattern of Gilles de la Tourette syndrome is fluid and symptoms may vary in severity from week to week. Some particular problem may disappear for a time, only to reappear again at a later date.

Remissions can occur in some children, but usually the motor and vocal tics and the obsessive behaviour will reassert themselves again after a brief interval.

MANAGEMENT IMPLICATIONS

Various drugs have been, and are still being, tried to reduce the motor and vocal tics. Results have been variable, but some success has been possible.

Schooling can be an especially difficult problem, due both to lack of concentration and to the difficult obsessive behaviour and repetitive multiple tics. Education may be necessary in a small unit where a variety of difficult behaviour patterns can be contained. It is of vital importance that the teaching staff are made aware of the diagnosis, so that appropriate care and teaching methods can be employed.

THE FUTURE

Gilles de la Tourette syndrome is not a life-threatening disorder, but normal career prospects can be markedly limited by the symptoms. Social contact is also difficult, or even impossible, if the sufferer is severely affected.

SELF-HELP GROUP

Tourette Syndrome (UK) Association
Valley Mead
27 Monckton Street
Ryde
Isle of Wight PO33 2BY
(Tel. 01983 568866)

Aims and provisions: support and contact between individuals and families; promotion of research; newsletter and booklets.

Goldenhar syndrome

ALTERNATIVE NAMES

Goldenhar-Gorlin syndrome; ocular-auriculo-vertebral anomaly; first and second branchial arch syndrome.

INCIDENCE

Studies on the incidence of this syndrome have only been recorded in the USA. In the Midwest of America one report observed an incidence of one in every 5600 live births. A further study reported an incidence of one in every 26 000 live births in the USA. There appears to be a slightly higher incidence of this syndrome in boys than in girls.

CAUSATION

Patterns of inheritance seem to vary, and both an autosomal dominant and an autosomal recessive inheritance appear to be possible. The effects of the manifestations of this syndrome vary greatly, even within the same family. This makes both accurate diagnosis and the sorting out of inheritance patterns difficult.

Ultra-sound examination antenatally may detect ear abnormalities if they are present and severe. Other skeletal abnormalities, including the small lower jaw, may also be visualized.

CHARACTERISTICS

Ears: Abnormalities in the anatomy of both the external and the middle ear are among the most obvious and important features. The size and shape of the external ear varies greatly ranging from virtually no external ear at all to a much misshapen pinna. This can occur in one or both ears. The middle ear, containing those tiny bones vital for normal hearing, the ossicles, can also be tiny or misshapen. If these ossicles are small and/or misshapen, sound will not be conducted properly into the nerves of hearing and a conductive hearing loss will occur.

In conjunction with these abnormalities in the ear, the facial nerve can also occasionally run an unusual course. The Eustachian tube, linking the middle ear to the back of the throat, is also sometimes malformed. These defects can all add to the hearing problem.

Asymmetry of the face is a further feature in well over half of the babies born with this syndrome. The asymmetry becomes more evident as the baby matures, and by the age of around four years the unusual shape of the child's face is very obvious.

Cleft palate, with occasionally a coexistent cleft lip, can add to the unusual facial features at birth.

A **small, receding chin** can also be a characteristic. If this is present, difficulties with feeding can be worrying in the early days of life.

Eyes may be small with narrowing of the actual eyelids, making the eyes appear even smaller. About one-third of children with Goldenhar's syndrome have pinkish, yellowish growths, often containing much fatty tissue, in their eyes. These can grow to be as big as 10 mm in diameter. When they reach this size, vision can become obscured.

Other **skeletal abnormalities** can be present and wide-ranging, varying from unusually shaped vertebrae, which will eventually give rise to scoliosis, to abnormalities in the forearm and thumbs. (These latter features are reminiscent of the abnormalities seen in both the CHARGE and VATER associations. These two 'associations' of anomalies have somewhat similar defects in the forearm region. There is, however, no connection between these conditions and the Goldenhar syndrome.)

Heart defects occur with greater frequency than in other babies. Reports as to the incidence of this type of abnormality varies. Some authorities put the incidence as high as 58% of babies born with the Goldenhar syndrome. Ventricular septal defects are reported as being one of the most common of these heart abnormalities.

In a few children with this syndrome there may be some degree of **learning disability**. Also, some children with very deformed faces can have severe **emotional** problems.

MANAGEMENT IMPLICATIONS

In the early days of life, feeding can be a problem if the baby has a tiny lower jaw (cf Pierre–Robin syndrome). If there is also a cleft palate, with or without an associated cleft lip, this will add to the feeding difficulties. Tube feeding may be necessary in the early days to ensure adequate nutrition. The most severe cases can need surgical intervention for feeds to be given directly into the stomach. The unusual facial features can also lead to breathing difficulties, especially during sleep. A tiny lower jaw can allow the tongue to fall back into the throat, thereby obstructing breathing. Babies should be put to sleep on their sides to avoid this.

Hearing loss must also be diagnosed and fully assessed as early in life as possible to minimize the risk of delayed speech. The maximum age for the acquisition of speech and language is usually between one and two years. But before this time the baby is gathering information regarding various sound patterns by listening, especially to his/her parents. Any loss of hearing at either of these important stages can result in a much delayed speech ability. Once the hearing loss is diagnosed and treated as far as is possible, **speech therapy** is valuable and often necessary for clear, understandable speech. As well as problems due to hearing, children with the Goldenhar syndrome can have difficulties in articulating their words, due to their unusual facial features. Speech therapists have many methods of overcoming all these problems.

Eyes: if the typical growths are present in the eye region, they should be removed before their increasing size further precludes vision. Unfortunately, vision can also be adversely affected after this removal due to the scar tissue which inevitably forms following surgery.

Cleft palate will need surgical repair if this defect is present. Surgery may also be needed for other facial asymmetries if they are severe and amenable to this form of treatment.

Dental care is also important following the eruption of the teeth. Due to the asymmetry of the face, teeth will not always meet together properly, so orthodontic care will be necessary.

Heart defects, if present, will need assessment and possible treatment depending on the type and effects the defect is having on the child.

Mental abilities will need to be checked by routine developmental assessment at regular intervals and assessment will need to be continued during the school years. Problems in any specific areas can thus be isolated and appropriate help given.

Emotional problems can arise particularly during the adolescent years if the facial disfigurement is very marked. Sensitive counselling and support from relatives and friends should reduce the impact of such problems to a minimum. Joining a group of similarly affected people can also do much to help.

THE FUTURE

Lifespan is not restricted unless heart defects are severe or not amenable to treatment. Careers may be limited in choice if there is any substantial hearing loss. Facial disfigurement may also be a factor precluding careers much in the public eye.

Genetic counselling when pregnancy is being considered is advisable.

SELF-HELP GROUPS

Goldenhar Syndrome Support Group
23 Eldon Street
Greenock
Renfrewshire
Scotland PA16 7UG
(Tel. 01475 781263)

Aims and provisions: support and contact with other affected families; information leaflets.

'Let's Face It' (network for the facially disfigured)
10 Wood End
Crowthorne
Berkshire RG11 6DQ
(Tel. 01344 774405)

This organization will also give support to people with facial disfigurements of all kinds.

Guillain Barre syndrome

ALTERNATIVE NAME

Infective polyneuritis.

INCIDENCE

The true incidence of Guillain Barre syndrome is not known. There have been suggestions that the incidence in children has increased over the past two decades. The commonest time for the condition to occur seems to be in children between the ages of four and ten, although Guillain Barre syndrome is not unknown in babies. Both boys and girls appear to be equally affected.

CAUSATION

There has been much discussion over the years regarding the cause of the Guillain Barre syndrome. As the condition frequently follows on from an acute infection it has been thought that it may be due to the toxic effects of this original infection. Hypersensitivity to some substance or organism, or the reactivation of a latent virus, have been other suggestions as to the cause.

There is no inheritance pattern involved in Guillain Barre syndrome.

CHARACTERISTICS

Guillain Barre syndrome will often start with **tingling** in the hands and feet. Along with these sensations will go severe pains in the legs together with tenderness when muscles are touched. This latter symptom is due to inflammation of the sensory nerves. All these symptoms can be of varying severity, ranging from acute pain to only intermittent tingling sensations.

Within a few days, legs will become markedly weak, and walking will be difficult. This weakness gradually extends up the body to the arms and, most serious of all, to the muscles involved with respiration. The young sufferer will feel generally unwell, and may have a mild fever, although this is often not a feature.

Symptoms will persist and may worsen for around a week or two, during which time the child is gravely ill. Admission to hospital is necessary and artificial ventilation may be needed to maintain breathing. Muscles around the face and throat can also become involved, making swallowing difficult or impossible.

Once this acute stage is over, recovery begins. This is slow and can take many months before the young sufferer is fully fit again and able to use weakened muscles fully. Recovery is usually complete and only a very small minority of children are left with any residual weakness. If this does occur, the disability is only minimal.

MANAGEMENT IMPLICATIONS

Acute stage: once the diagnosis has been made, urgent admission to hospital is necessary. Intensive therapy facilities need to be readily available to ensure that respiration is maintained. There is no specific treatment available, reliance being placed on good nursing care, and maintenance of respiration should this become necessary.

Convalescence can be long, with paralysed muscles only slowly returning to full use. During this time, children will need adequate rest, a good diet and plenty of quiet pastimes available. Later on in convalescence schoolwork can be sent home so that too much schooling is not missed.

THE FUTURE

Guillain Barre syndrome is a serious illness, but fortunately the outlook in the long-term is good with little or no permanent sequelae.

SELF-HELP GROUP

British Guillain Barre Support Group
'Foxley'
Holdingham
Sleaford
Lincolnshire NG34 8NR
(Tel. 01529 304615

Aims and provisions: emotional support for people during recovery; public awareness about the disease; leaflets and other publications available.

Haemolytic-uraemic syndrome

INCIDENCE

This is a rare syndrome, but one which can arise in clusters in different parts of the country. There are two quite separate ways in which this syndrome can arise, one of which is inherited and the other probably arising as the result of a viral infection. The exact occurrence is not known, but over 100 families having a member with the condition have been recorded. Either sex can be affected.

CAUSATION

The hereditary form of this syndrome arises as either an autosomal dominant or an autosomal recessive condition. This inherited causative factor is thought to account for only about 5% of the known cases.

Other children, and adults, can suffer from the haemolytic-uraemic syndrome as a result of a previous acute gastro-intestinal illness. It can be difficult to distinguish the hereditary form of this syndrome from the acquired type, but there are two specific features which can point to one or other of the causative factors. First, in the acquired form of the haemolytic-uraemic syndrome, symptoms of severe gastro-enteritis with bloody diarrhoea, and perhaps vomiting, are the early features of the condition. In the case of the inherited form, there is rarely any such preceding gastric upset – the characteristic features arising 'out of the blue'. Secondly, with the acquired type, other family members may go down with a similar illness within days or weeks of the first sufferer's illness. With the inherited form the interval between the onset of the illness in another related person can be anything between one and 14 years.

The haemolytic-uraemic syndrome can affect children (and adults) at any age from a few months onwards.

Whatever the causative factor, the features of the haemolytic-uraemic syndrome are similar, apart from the mode of onset.

CHARACTERISTICS

Following on from the acute gastro-intestinal infection seen in cases of presumably infective origin, the following features occur:

- **Anaemia** of a haemolytic type – the child will be pale, lethargic, feel unwell and tire readily on the slightest exertion. On checking the blood, the red blood cells are seen to be distorted and fragmented, and hence lose much of their haemoglobin (the oxygen-carrying substance in the red blood cells). The platelet count is also often extremely low. (Platelets are intimately concerned with the clotting of the blood.) Haemorrhages under the skin can arise as a result of these blood changes.
- **Renal failure** can develop rapidly. Urine output may be much reduced, or there may be no urine passed at all. What urine is passed is seen to be bloodstained. The child is acutely and seriously ill, with perhaps very much raised blood pressure and cardiac failure. He/she will be restless and confused and convulsions can occur. Death can result during this very serious acute phase of the illness.

The pathology behind these serious events is thought to be damage to the tiny blood vessels walls inside the kidneys. Following on from this, the blood cells are themselves damaged as a result of the rough, damaged blood vessel walls. A defect in the metabolism of a specific chemical, prostacyclin, has been suggested to be the prime cause of the haemolytic-uraemic syndrome.

Following on from the acute illness, damage to the central nervous system (probably as a result of the convulsions which can occur) may occur, resulting in a residual **learning disability**. This is by no means always the case, but must be remembered as a possibility. A recurrence of the acute illness can occur in some children at a later date. This particular occurrence is thought only to happen in those people who suffer from the haemolytic-uraemic syndrome which arises as a recessively inherited characteristic.

Treatment is dialysis to combat the acute renal failure. Blood transfusion will also be necessary to treat the haemolytic anaemia. This must be given with care in order not to overload the circulation, with the concomitant damaged renal output, with fluid.

Chronic renal failure may be the unfortunate end result if the acute stage of the disease is survived. This may require repeated haemodialysis, or continuous peritoneal dialysis. Kidney transplantation is the best long-term outlook.

MANAGEMENT IMPLICATIONS

The **acute** stage of the haemolytic-uraemic syndrome will need intensive care facilities in hospital to combat the renal failure and possible hypertension and cardiac failure. Any succeeding recurrences of the condition will also need to be treated in a similar way.

Continuous ambulatory peritoneal dialysis may be the best way to treat a child with chronic renal failure following acute illness, whilst he/she is awaiting renal transplantation. Children accept this necessary treatment surprisingly well and become adept at coping with their unusual excretory process.

Learning disability following the acute illness must be recognized and subjected to detailed assessment. Some few children may require special educational facilities. If this is the case, on-going assessment and help must be given.

THE FUTURE

The outlook for sufferers from the haemolytic-uraemic syndrome is not good for those with the inherited form. In one report, between 70% and 90% were found to have died as a result of their illness and 6% of the survivors were in chronic renal failure. Further attacks of acute illness may also occur.

Survivors of the acquired type may also suffer from chronic renal failure or, conversely, may make a complete recovery.

Career prospects will depend on the amount of residual disability. Life expectancy will also depend on the severity of the after-effects. Genetic counselling is indicated particularly in those families in whom there is more than one member with the condition.

SELF-HELP GROUP

There is no specific self-help group associated with the haemolytic uraemic syndrome, but the following organization can give reliable help and advice for renal problems:

British Kidney Patient Association
Bordon
Hampshire
(Tel. 01420 472021)

Haemophilia

ALTERNATIVE NAMES

Classic haemophilia; factor 8 deficiency; haemophilia A.

INCIDENCE

The incidence of this well-known inherited condition is one in every 10 000
live male births (only boys are affected, due to the mode of inheritance).
All races can be affected.

Haemophilia is a descriptive name used to describe a number of blood
disorders which all have clotting problems as the basic defect. There are
a number of 'factors' associated with the clotting mechanism of the blood.
Haemophilia A is specifically deficient in factor 8. Other factors are
involved in the clotting disorders of other similar diseases, such as Christmas disease and Von Willebrand's disease.

HISTORY

Haemophilia has been known for many years, and is well-documented in
history. Effective treatment was not available until the early 1960s. Previous to this, haemophilia was often fatal in childhood, or led to much
disability and a restricted lifestyle.

CAUSATION

Haemophilia A has an X-linked recessive inheritance. There is an abnormal factor 8 molecule in sufferers from this condition, leading to the
abnormal clotting mechanism. Between one-fifth and one-third of all cases

are thought to arise sporadically as new mutations. The disease can be mild, moderate or severe. It is thought that there may be a different type of genetic inheritance in these three manifestations of the disease. About half of all known cases of classic haemophilia have the severe form of the disease. About 80% of sufferers have positive family history of haemophilia. The condition can be diagnosed antenatally by fetoscopy.

CHARACTERISTICS

All the features of haemophilia are entirely due to the defective clotting mechanism. The condition can be diagnosed at birth. Excessive bleeding from the umbilical cord can be the first clue as to the possibility of a bleeding disorder.

In severely affected boys, **haemorrhages** into joints are common. This occurs following only minimal trauma, or may be nothing more than the usual vigorous movements of joints common to all active children. Hips, knees and ankles in the lower limbs can all be affected as can wrists and elbows in particular in the upper limbs. This leads to **painful, swollen joints**, the excess blood inside the capsules of the joints causing the pain. Appropriate treatment must be given early to avoid damage and eventual destruction of the affected joints. Before the advent of specific treatment, grossly deformed joints due to degenerative arthritis was the inevitable result of frequent haemorrhagic incidents. This was especially evident in the weight-bearing joints such as hips and knees.

Bruising in soft tissues all over the body is commonly seen in haemophiliac boys. Again this results from only minor bumps.

In young children, bleeding from minor injuries to the **tongue** and **lips** is common. During the early days of learning to walk, falls are common and are often associated with damage to the mouth region. Inadvertent biting of the tongue is also common when learning to cope with solid food. Both these everyday events can lead to severe haemorrhage in the boy with haemophilia.

Bumps on the **head** are again very common during the growing years. This can result in disastrous bleeding into the brain unless rapid treatment is given. This is one of the major causes of death in the young child with haemophilia.

Less severely affected children will not be so vulnerable to minor injury. It is only when surgery (for tonsillectomy and other relatively minor procedures, for example) is undertaken that the clotting defect is a problem. The more serious injuries, such as those caused in road accidents, that can be sustained by any child, will also result in severe bleeding.

In cases of suspected child abuse, the possibility of haemophilia – if not already known – must always be remembered.

Haemophiliac boys are especially susceptible to infection with **hepatitis B**. This can lead to progressive liver disease with a potentially fatal outcome. As soon as the diagnosis of haemophilia is made, immunization against hepatitis B should be given.

Treatment is by the administering factor 8. Prompt infusion of this compound will limit the damage done by bleeding into joints. The treatment must be given as soon as the bleeding occurs. Some boys with haemophilia will develop a specific 'inhibitor', or immunity, to routine treatment. Subsequent haemorrhagic events will then need to be treated at a specialized haemophiliac centre. Some years ago, blood products used to treat haemophiliac patients were, regrettably, contaminated with HIV and a number of sufferers have succumbed to AIDS as a result. Heat-treated products, which render HIV non-infectious, are now used for treatment.

MANAGEMENT IMPLICATIONS

It can be difficult to strike the correct balance in a boy with haemophilia between over-protection and lack of restraint. Parents will feel they must avoid even the slightest injury to their son with the resultant probability of severe haemorrhage. On the other hand, the child must be allowed to explore and investigate his environment as part of the growing process. It is all too easy for the boy with haemophilia to develop **emotional problems** as a result of his genetic inheritance. Support and advice from doctors, nurses and other professionals experienced in the handling of children with haemophilia is important.

Parents become very experienced during the early years in assessing the significance of any injury, and will also become adept at giving the appropriate treatment.

Schooling will obviously present greater risks to the haemophiliac child. Teachers must be fully conversant with the action to be taken if a knock or other injury results in a bleed into a joint or other tissues. The telephone number of the haemophiliac centre responsible for the treatment of the child should be available in school. If in any doubt as to the action to be taken following an injury, advice can be obtained from this source.

Contact sports and other violent physical activities must not be part of the curriculum for the haemophiliac boy.

Education has an important part to play in the future career of a boy with this condition. Manual work cannot be contemplated, so intellectual pursuits and careers are of vital importance.

Care should also be taken in the use of aspirin in haemophiliac boys due to the possibility of Reye's syndrome occurring in a small number of children.

VON WILLEBRAND'S DISEASE (OR PSEUDO-HAEMOPHILIA)

This is a condition which also has a relative deficiency in factor 8. Unlike haemophilia A, Von Willebrand's disease can affect both boys and girls, as the inheritance pattern is either an autosomal dominant or an autosomal recessive.

Symptoms of bleeding are much less pronounced than in haemophilia A. Nevertheless, epistaxis (nosebleed) is common and bruising on minimal injury can result. In girls excessive menstrual flow can be a problem resulting in much discomfort and possibly in anaemia. Excessive bleeding following surgery can also be a problem.

Treatment is by administering cryoprecipitate factor 8. Immunization against hepatitis B is also a wise precaution.

Later in life care must be taken in women to control bleeding following childbirth.

THE FUTURE

With adequate quick treatment of bleeding episodes, the outlook is good nowadays for haemophiliac boys. Careers which include physical activities must be avoided, and contact sports must not be indulged in.

SELF-HELP GROUP

The Haemophiliac Society
123 Westminster Bridge Road
London SEX 7HR
(Tel. 0171 928 2020)

This group will be able to give advice and support.

Homocystinuria

INCIDENCE

Homocystinuria is one of the rare metabolic diseases. As with other meta-bolic conditions, knowledge of the biochemical nature of the problem has vastly increased over the past decade. As a result of the screening programmes on new-born babies in most parts of the world, it has been found that Ireland appears to have one of the highest incidences of homo-cystinuria. In this country one in 60 000 babies are likely to be affected, whereas in Japan the number of babies with this particular metabolic problem has been estimated to be as low as one in 146 000. Both boys and girls can be affected.

CAUSATION

Homocystinuria is inherited as an autosomal recessive condition.

CHARACTERISTICS

Homocystinuria is a defect in the enzyme metabolism of specific amino acids – homocystine and methionine. Excess homocystine is excreted in the urine and both homocystine and methionine can be found in excess in the plasma.

These two facts form the basis of the biochemical diagnosis and also result in several features.

Skeletal system: children with homocytinuria are usually tall with long, slender fingers. (This, together with the eye problems, are very much the same features as are found in Marfan's syndrome.) Scoliosis may also be present, as well as knock-knees and chest deformities.

Eyes are commonly affected in homocystinuria, dislocation of the lens being the most common abnormality. Short-sight is also common and glaucoma and retinal detachment are further complications that can occur later in life. Appropriate treatment when, and if, these complications occur can reduce the incidence of severe visual problems.

Blood system: effects on the vascular system are the most worrying aspects of homocystinuria. Thromboses occur with greater frequency than normal and can occur anywhere in the body – brain, heart or eyes, for example. Symptoms will occur in relationship to the part of the vascular system that is affected. (Due to this, venepuncture and surgical procedures should be avoided if at all possible, or certainly undertaken with great care.) This abnormal clotting can occur at any time of life, including infancy and childhood. The exact mechanism of this phenomenon is not fully understood.

Central nervous system: most homocystinuria sufferers have normal mental abilities, but a minority can show mild to moderate learning disability. Early treatment does seem to help mitigate this. If thrombosis has occurred in the brain, this may also have a deleterious effect on mental abilities as well as the physical neurological signs. Convulsions can also occur, although this is comparatively rare and, again, can be helped by appropriate treatment.

MANAGEMENT IMPLICATIONS

Some cases of homocystinuria can be helped by treatment with vitamin B6 (pyridoxin), many features of the disease being improved; it is of vital importance that the susceptibility to treatment with pyridoxin is determined early so that various manifestations of the condition can be alleviated. The vitamin is given on a regular basis and levels of the relevant amino acids in the blood are measured regularly. If these levels approach normal limits, treatment is continued throughout life with, of course, regular monitoring.

Folic acid supplements also appear to be necessary in some people with homocystinuria. This maximizes the good effects of the vitamin B6. A diet low in methionine can also be valuable, and the help of a dietitian is of great value under these circumstances.

Eyes: visual acuity must be assessed regularly and corrective lenses prescribed for any refractive error found. The increased possibility of glaucoma and retinal detachment must also be borne in mind.

Vascular system: any thrombotic episodes, with the possible damaging sequelae, must be managed medically as they occur.

Central nervous system: children should receive regular developmental checks, with monitoring continuing when school-age is reached. Appropriate schooling can then be arranged should any problems be found. Checking of intellectual abilities after any central nervous system thrombotic episodes is also advisable.

THE FUTURE

With appropriate early treatment in the vitamin B6–responsive type of homocytinuria, the outlook is good and life expectancy is normal. Vitamin B6–unresponsive cases will have to rely on dietary measures as the sole form of available treatment. Under these circumstances, life-threatening thromboses are more likely to occur, but research is showing that early dietary restrictions, conscientiously adhered to throughout life, does improve the outlook.

Due to the increased risk of thrombosis it is not advisable for oral contraceptives to be used.

SELF-HELP GROUP

There is no specific self-help group, but the following offers help, support and advice to all sufferers of metabolic disease and their families:

Research Trust for Metabolic Disease in Children (RTMDC)
Golden Gates Lodge
Weston Road
Crewe
Cheshire CW1 1XN
(Tel. 01270 250221)

Hunter's syndrome

ALTERNATIVE NAME

Mucopolysaccharidosis 2.

INCIDENCE

Hunter's syndrome is an example of a defect in the metabolism of the complex sugars – the mucopolysaccharides. There are a number of syndromes in this group, and in each there is lack of a specific enzyme which controls the metabolism of these nutrients (Other syndromes include Hurler's syndrome, Morquio's syndrome and San Filippo syndrome.) Around one in 100 000 live births exhibit Hunter's syndrome. Due to the mode of inheritance of Hunter's syndrome, only boys have been known to be affected. All races of the world appear to have the possibility of being affected.

HISTORY

Until relatively recently, only seven mucopolysaccharide syndromes had been described – each due to a different enzyme defect. Recently however, 11 variants have been found, each with defective metabolism of a complex sugar. It is possible that further similar enzyme defects can occur.

CAUSATION

Hunter's syndrome is inherited in an X-linked recessive way, so no girls are seen with Hunter's syndrome. Mothers carrying the characteristics can pass them onto their sons. The enzyme involved in Hunter's syndrome is a complicated one known as iduronate sulphatase. Due to the deficiency of this enzyme, mucopolysaccharides (complex sugars) accumulate in the organs and tissues of the body, where they give rise to the typical signs and symptoms of the syndrome.

Hunter's syndrome can be detected at around the ninth week of pregnancy by chorionic villus sampling techniques.

CHARACTERISTICS

There are two types of Hunter's syndrome – one of which is milder and runs a less progressively downhill course than the more severe type.

These two types can be distinguished biochemically by the complex sugar which is excreted in the urine. It is the accumulation of this specific sugar in the organs and tissues which gives rise to the following characteristics.

Boys with Hunter's syndrome appear to have no problems at birth. They grow normally and pass all their developmental milestones at the proper time. During these early days the only noticeable problem can be noisy breathing, which is frequently associated with a blocked and runny nose. But as this is often part of normal childhood anyway, no-one's attention is drawn to other possible problems. Head circumference measurements are within the upper limits of normal during these early years.

Umbilical, or inguinal, **hernias** are more frequently seen in babies who are subsequently found to have Hunter's syndrome, than is usual. But once again, boys not having Hunter's syndrome can also have these weaknesses in the abdominal wall and so attention is not alerted.

From around two years of age onwards there is an obvious coarsening of the **facial features**. The boy's neck will be short, and his erupting teeth will be seen to be coming through widely spaced. Also over the succeeding months, these features are combined with a slowing down of the growth rate.

Joints can become stiff and the body is also often seen to be covered with a fine, downy **hair**.

At this time the **liver** and **spleen** become enlarged as a direct result of the accumulation of mucopolysaccarides in these organs. This enlargement can be a factor in the onset – or recurrence – of umbilical herniae.

Mentally, children with the mild form of Hunter's syndrome are of normal intelligence or only very mildly disabled. Unfortunately, with the severe form, learning disability is greater and will be obvious by around the age of eight to ten years.

As the boy matures, deposits of mucopolysaccharides can be found in many organs of the body – heart valves, coronary arteries, meninges and joints all being possibly included. It is one, or more, of these complications that will result in an illness with maybe a fatal outcome in a boy with Hunter's syndrome. For instance, the damage to heart valves and/or coronary arteries gives rise to heart failure or, in the case of a blocked coronary artery, sudden death.

This clinical picture is very similar to that seen in the other mucopolysaccharidoses, although the basic genetic and biochemical faults are different.

MANAGEMENT IMPLICATIONS

There is, regrettably, no curative treatment for Hunter's syndrome. Parents need sensitive counselling as to the future of their son, it being important to lay emphasis on the help that can be given to make life as normal as possible for their child – and themselves.

Herniae: if this weakness of the abdominal wall is present, this must be dealt with surgically. But (as in Hurler's syndrome), there is a high likelihood of recurrence due to further accumulations of mucopolysaccharides which increase the pressure inside the abdominal wall, pushing the contents into weakened areas.

Hearing must be checked on a regular basis for children with Hunter's syndrome. Distraction tests suitable to the mental age of the boy will need to be done. Pure-tone audiometry is a further option, with evoked responses as a further aid to diagnosis where necessary. Deafness is common and hearing aids may be necessary later in childhood.

Contractures of joints, which can lead to grossly limited movement, can be kept to a minimum by physiotherapy. Hydrotherapy is particularly valuable and soothing. Therapy should be on-going, with parents being involved in the treatment of their son as far as is possible. Sometimes surgery may be necessary to correct joint deformities.

Learning disability in the severe type of Hunter's syndrome will need special education. Regular developmental checks are necessary to monitor all aspects of on-going development in the boy with Hunter's syndrome. The results of such monitoring are necessary when decisions are being made as to the need, or otherwise, for special educational facilities.

With the milder type of Hunter's syndrome, normal schooling is usually satisfactory.

THE FUTURE

Children with the severe type of Hunter's syndrome often only survive into their mid-teens to twenties. Cardiac problems, or severe respiratory infection, is the usual cause of death in the early or mid twenties.

Boys with the milder type of Hunter's syndrome enjoy a longer lifespan, and sufferers have been known to survive into their late sixties.

Children have been born to fathers with Hunter's syndrome. Families who have a boy with Hunter's syndrome will need genetic counselling. Girls carrying the defective gene can be identified and this is of crucial importance when pregnancy is being considered.

SELF-HELP GROUP

Society for Mucopolysaccharide Diseases
55 Hill Avenue
Amersham
Buckinghamshire HP6 5BX
(Tel. 01494 434156)

Aims and provisions: support and advice for parents; raise funds for research; annual parent conference held.

Hurler's syndrome

ALTERNATIVE NAMES

Gargoylism; mucopolysaccharidosis 1–H.

INCIDENCE

Hurler's syndrome is one of a group of diseases known as the mucopolysaccharidoses. These conditions are all similar in that they all owe their characteristics to accumulations of mucopolysaccharides (complex sugars), in the tissues of the body. Enzymes necessary to the breakdown of these complex sugars are defective in these conditions. The enzyme responsible differs in each syndrome of this group.

All the mucopolysaccharide diseases differ clinically, genetically and biochemically from each other. There are probably up to 11 different mucopolysaccharide abnormalities. (See Hunter's syndrome, Morquio's syndrome and San Filippo syndrome. The remaining syndromes in this group are exceedingly rare.) Around one in 10 000 live births exhibit Hurler's syndrome. The sexes are equally represented and Hurler's syndrome has been described in all races.

HISTORY

The mucopolysaccharidoses have been known for some time, but until recent years the specific enzyme defect in each type had not been isolated. Classification has also been a problem in the past, but this has now been standardized.

CAUSATION

Hurler's syndrome is caused by a genetic defect inherited as an autosomal recessive. The particular enzyme which is deficient in Hurler's syndrome is alpha-L-iduronidase. This deficiency results in high levels of mucopolysaccharides being both excreted in the urine and deposited in the tissues.

Hurler's syndrome can be detected antenatally by assay of the specific enzyme from chorionic villus sampling and also by amniocentesis.

CHARACTERISTICS

Children with Hurler's syndrome appear to be normal at birth, although they may be very **large babies**, but from the early months of life onward the following features will appear.

Facial features will gradually become coarsened, with a depressed nasal bridge, a large tongue, large lips and widely spaced teeth. Along with these features goes a persistently blocked and runny nose associated also with noisy breathing.

Abdominally, a **large spleen and liver** may be felt and also seen. Many toddlers do normally have big tummies due to the relatively large size of the liver at this age. But the child with Hurler's syndrome will show this to excess. Also, the usual 'slimming down' of the late pre-school years will not occur; instead the large abdomen will increase in size. By two years of age there is frequently a large umbilical and/or inguinal hernia present. This is due to the increased pressure of the abdominal organs, which are very much enlarged by the accumulation of mucopolysaccharides.

Skeletal system: many joints become stiff and eventually lose much of their range of mobility altogether, unless steps are taken to correct this. The spine can become curved in both the upper and lower back regions; the former eventually giving rise to a grossly deformed chest. By two years of age, the child will be noticeably shorter than his contemporaries. This is due to the lack of growth, which had been normal up to between six to 18 months, but which thereafter proceeds only very slowly.

Eyes: the cornea becomes progressively clouded after the first few months of life. Eventually vision becomes very limited due both to the corneal clouding and also to degenerative changes in the retina.

Learning disability: as the child matures, deposits of mucopolysaccharides accumulate in the brain. This leads to a variable degree of learning disability. Many children will lose some of the skills they have already learned.

Cardiac defects can arise at any time. Once again, this is due to deposits of mucopolysaccharides in the heart and coronary arteries. As the valves and walls of the coronary arteries become infiltrated, signs of heart failure can occur – breathlessness, swelling of lower limbs and lassitude, for example.

There is a further variant of Hurler's syndrome, known as Scheie syndrome (mucopolysaccharidosis AS), which also has a deficiency of the same enzyme as that in Hurler's syndrome. Characteristics are similar to those seen in Hurler's syndrome, but are fortunately much milder. There is also a similar genetic inheritance.

MANAGEMENT IMPLICATIONS

Once the diagnosis has been made (by biochemical findings of reduced enzyme activity, elevation of specific mucopolysaccharides and specific X-ray appearances in bones) plans will need to be made to care for a child who will have increasing disability, both mental and physical. Parents must be sensitively counselled as to the likely outcome of their child's genetic problem.

Umbilical and/or inguinal herniae will need surgery both to prevent the possibility of strangulation and for the child's comfort. Due to the continuing progressive accumulation of mucopolysaccharides, both these conditions may recur and need further treatment.

Stiff joints may also need surgical help, but physiotherapy – most helpful in warm water – will give symptomatic relief. Children much enjoy this form of therapy.

Heart abnormalities need to be monitored closely by way of cardiac function. Surgical treatment may be found to be necessary, but has not proved to be of long-lasting value due to the continuing nature of the underlying problem.

Learning disability, **visual difficulties** and **deafness**, again all due to progressive deposition of mucopolysaccharides, will need special educational facilities eventually. Frequent assessment of possible deterioration of vision and hearing as well as mental abilities is necessary, so that the child with Hurler's syndrome can be cared for in an optimum environment. Methods of communication other than vision or hearing may need to be learned if usual methods of communication become a problem.

It is probable that the child with Hurler's syndrome will become wheelchair bound eventually. Special facilities in the child's home and school for toileting, bathing and other activities will then be necessary.

THE FUTURE

Regrettably, as Hurler's syndrome is a progressive disorder for which there is no cure at present, life expectancy is poor. Few children reach their teens. Death is usually due either to pneumonia following the frequent respiratory illness or to heart failure.

Enzyme replacement therapy has been tried to no avail. At present, bone-marrow transplants are being evaluated.

SELF-HELP GROUPS

The Society for Mucopolysaccharide Diseases
55 Hill Avenue
Amersham
Buckinghamshire HP6 5BX
(Tel. 01494 434156)

Aims and provisions: support and advice for families; raises funds for research; annual parent weekend conference held.

Disabled Living Foundation
246 Kensington High Street
London

This group is also a useful contact point for special equipment.

Hypertrophic cardio-myopathy

ALTERNATIVE NAMES

Muscular sub-aortic stenosis; hypertrophic obstructive cardio-myopathy.

INCIDENCE

The exact incidence of this condition is not known, but is thought to be around one in 10 000. (It will probably never be possible to determine the exact incidence of hypertrophic cardio-myopathy. Many people are unaware that they have this cardiac abnormality as they never have any symptoms throughout life. One of the aims of the self-help group concerned with this condition is to try and establish more clearly just how many people in the UK are affected.) Its importance lies in the fact that sudden death can occur, even in young people, if the disease has not been recognized.

The condition has been reported from all over the world in people of all races. Both sexes are equally affected.

HISTORY

Hypertrophic cardio-myopathy was first recognized as a specific heart defect in the late 1950s.

CAUSATION

It is thought that this heart problem is inherited as an autosomal dominant condition. Once a diagnosis has been made in one family member it is strongly recommended that the remainder of first-degree relatives (parents, children, brothers, sisters) should be screened for the condition.

Reports of abnormalities in the genes on chromosome 14 in some families with hypertrophic cardio-myopathy have been received. Work is proceeding on the genetics of this condition.

CHARACTERISTICS

The basic abnormality in the hearts of people with hypertrophic cardio-myopathy is a thickening in the wall of some part of the ventricles (the 'pumping' chambers of the heart) – usually the left – or the septum dividing the two sides of the heart. When looked at under the microscope the cells in the abnormal part of the heart are seen to be randomly arranged instead of in the symmetrical pattern seen in normal heart muscle. The overall effect of this abnormality is to reduce the pumping action of the heart. In addition to this, two further effects can occur:

- The 'disarray' in the heart muscle can interfere with the normal electrical conducting mechanism controlling the rhythm of the heart;
- if the thickened part of the heart is high in the septum this can interfere with the action of the mitral valve. This valve controls the blood flow between the left ventricle and left atrium. (The atria of the heart are the two upper 'collecting' chambers of the heart.)

Although this condition is probably present at birth in most cases, it is usually not until the teenage or early adult years that symptoms begin to occur. The reason why the condition becomes apparent – by the following symptoms – at this time is unclear.

Breathlessness on any unusual exertion is often one of the first signs of problems. The teenager will not be able to keep up with peers in competitive games or cross-country running, for example. Alternatively the sufferer may suddenly take a dislike to all forms of extra physical exercise, not liking to admit to becoming unduly breathless. (This symptom is so often correlated with advancing age!)

Chest pain can also be a warning sign. The pain is felt centrally in the chest and is often made worse by exercise, although it can occur when sitting quietly. The reason for this pain is probably a lack of sufficient oxygen for the thickened muscles to work properly.

Palpitations, in which the heart beat is irregular, and often most uncomfortably at a fast rate. At times these irregularities can lead to feelings of **light-headedness, dizziness** and occasionally to **loss of consciousness**. The risk of sudden death is greater in people with this condition than for those with completely normal hearts.

Endocarditis – an infection of the inner lining of the heart – is also a risk associated with this condition. This is due to the greater ability of bacteria, present in the blood-stream in generalized infections, to stick to the roughened lining of the heart. This roughness occurs due to the turbulence of the blood-flow through the heart, which in turn, is due to the thickened walls.

All the above symptoms must be more fully investigated to determine the true cause. If hypertrophic cardio-myopathy is thought to be the cause further investigations will be necessary. (Only comparatively minor abnormalities can be heard through the stethoscope in this condition. For example, a forceful heart beat which is also transmitted to the pulses in wrist and neck. Also, if the mitral valve is involved there will be a typical 'murmur' to be heard.)

INVESTIGATIONS

An electro-cardiogram will be necessary to show abnormal electrical signals due to the disorganization of the cardiac muscle. However, in a few people with hypertrophic cardio-myopathy the ECG readings are normal. Under these latter circumstances – if the physical symptoms suggest that this disease is present – further investigations will be necessary, such as **echocardiography**. This is an ultra-sound scan of the heart and will readily show the thickened muscles if these are present. Doppler ultra-sound can also be used to produce images of the blood-flow inside the heart as well as measuring its filling capacity.

There are also a number of other investigations that may need to be done to obtain a clear picture of what is going on inside the heart:

- **Cardiac catheterization**. This is an examination in which a fine tube is passed into the heart from a blood vessel in the leg. This is done X-ray guidance. This allows pressures inside the heart to be measured and blood-flow through the valves to be seen.
- **Continuous 24–hour ECG monitoring**. This is done by a small ECG machine being attached to the chest with a tape recorder in a small bag around the patient's waist. In this way a continuous record of the heart's action can be obtained. This shows the type and frequency of any arrhythmias.
- **Exercise tolerance tests**. Carefully graded exercise tests can also be a useful measure of heart function.

MANAGEMENT IMPLICATIONS

For many children and young people with this condition, its presence will not be known unless screening has taken place due to another family member found to be suffering from hyopertrophic cardio-myopathy. Even if the condition is known to be present, there may be no symptoms at all during early childhood. But care needs to be taken without over-protecting the child too much.

Exercise should only be undertaken within the limits of cardiac function. Children who become breathless or otherwise distressed after exercise should not be allowed to take part in strenuous games or competitive sports.

Drugs, of various kinds, are only necessary if heart dysfunctions are present. This must be decided upon and closely followed-up by both general practitioner and a cardiologist.

Antibiotics should be given prophylactically when any major dental work, such as the extraction of teeth, is undertaken. This is to minimize the risk of endocarditis.

Diet should be generally sensible, controlling excess weight. All people with this condition should be advised to avoid smoking

THE FUTURE

Genetic counselling is advisable before pregnancy is embarked upon, so that the risk of the baby being affected by the condition can be estimated. Pregnancy and labour can be entirely normal for the woman with hypertrophic cardio-myopathy. Pregnancy does, of course, impose an increased demand on the work of the heart and some women may have symptoms due to their heart condition for the first time during pregnancy. Others who have had symptoms already may find these worsening. Here again, specialist advice is necessary. Epidural anaesthesia during labour is best avoided as blood-pressure can drop excessively.

SELF-HELP GROUP

The Hypertrophic Cardio-myopathy Association
'Waverley'
Lodge Drive
Rickmansworth
Hertfordshire WD3 4PT
(Tel. 01923 896776)

Aims and provisions: provides accurate and up-to-date information on the condition; support for families.

Klinefelter's syndrome

ALTERNATIVE NAMES

Chromosome XXY.

INCIDENCE

The incidence of Klinefelter's syndrome is surprisingly high. From chromosomal studies on new-born babies, approximately one in every 500 boys have the typical chromosomal pattern. In institutions for adults with learning disability, around one in every 100 men are found to have this chromosomal abnormality.

HISTORY

The typical characteristics of this syndrome were first described by Drs Klinefelter and Albright in 1942.

CAUSATION

An extra X chromosome (normal sex chromosomes for males are XY, and for females XX) is the usual pattern. This is caused by a complex fault in the cell division of one of the parent's sex cells, either the ovum or the sperm, which go to form the new baby.

There is also a 'mosaic' form of Klinefelter's syndrome in which only some of the body cells have an XXY chromosome pattern, the remainder having the normal XY count. (There can also be more complex chromosomal abnormalities, the resultant chromosomal pattern being XXXY or even XXXXY, but these are unusual.)

Broadly speaking, the severity of the characteristics will depend on the number of cells in the body which have the abnormal chromosome pattern.

CHARACTERISTICS

At birth and during early childhood there is no obvious evidence of any abnormality, apart form the chance finding of the **testes** being smaller than is usual. It is at puberty that the following changes become obvious.

The **testes** and **penis** of the boy with Klinefelter's syndrome are small. This decreased size of the sex organs persists into adult life when there is also a marked disturbance of sexual function. Infertility, impotence and decreased libido all result from this chromosomal abnormality. Blood testing shows increased levels of gonadotropins and a decreased level of testosterone.

A feminine type of **breast development** is also often obvious in boys with Klinefelter's syndrome.

Tall stature is also one of the consistent features of the syndrome. The body proportions are also unusual in as much as the legs are disproportionately long when compared with the trunk.

Body hair is usually scanty in boys with Klinefelter's syndrome. Normal pubic, axillary and chest hair fails to appear and daily shaving is rarely necessary.

Mental abilities are often at the low end of normal. Verbal skills seem to be especially affected in boys with Klinefelter's syndrome.

Psychological difficulties, due to the unusual sexual characteristics, are common when adolescence is reached. These persist into adult life and can merge into serious psychiatric problems.

Diabetes and **thyroid** problems are also more common than usual in boys and men with Klinefelter's syndrome.

MANAGEMENT IMPLICATIONS

The most serious effects of Klinefelter's syndrome are the **psychological trauma** felt by many boys at puberty when secondary sexual characteristics do not develop along normal lines. The testes and penis do not enlarge, pubic and axillary hair does not grow and breast development is more feminine than most boys would wish. Add to this, in many cases, slow mental ability and the scene is set for much psychological unhappiness. Boys will find ways to avoid the hurtful teasing to which they are frequently subjected and secondary behavioural problems often occur. For example the boy will often become the 'clown' of the class or will start to commit antisocial acts in an endeavour to gain the commendation of his peers in some way.

The help of a **clinical psychologist** can be of great value to the boy with Klinefelter's syndrome coming to terms with his genetic inheritance.

Testosterone therapy should be given from 11 to 12 years on. This will aid the development of more normal sexual characteristics, although it will have no effect on the infertility. But this treatment can help to reduce the psychological problems encountered during adolescence and early adult life.

Schooling: attendance at a mainstream school is usually possible for most boys with Klinefelter's syndrome, although some with more restricted intellectual abilities will need special facilities. The increased possibility of **diabetes** or **thyroid** imbalance must also be remembered.

THE FUTURE

All boys with Klinefelter's syndrome are infertile and only four men with the mosaic form of the syndrome have been known to father children.

Career choices may well be limited due to reduced mental abilities and also to the difficult behaviour found in some men and boys with this syndrome.

Life expectancy is thought to be normal.

SELF-HELP GROUPS

Klinefelter's Syndrome Association
56 Little Yeldham Road
Little Yeldham
Near Halstead
Essex
(Tel. 01787 237460)

Aims and provisions: contact with other families; support; information.

Teenage/Adult Contact
13 York Road
Orpington
Kent BR6 8PR
(Tel. 01689 70785)

Aims and provisions: support by letter; help with specific problems where possible.

Klippel–Feil syndrome

ALTERNATIVE NAMES

Klippel–Feil anomaly; congenital brevicollis; Klippel–Feil sequence, or disorder.

INCIDENCE

The reported incidence of Klippel–Feil syndrome is around one in 40 000 live births, girls being affected more than boys in an approximate ratio of 60 to 40. It is thought that many more children than this figure would suggest are mildly affected, but the abnormality is of such a mild degree as to pass unnoticed.

A number of different types of the condition have been described, depending on which part of the upper spine is most involved.

CAUSATION

Most cases of this syndrome are thought to arise sporadically but there are some reported families in which there are a number of affected individuals. These family histories point to an autosomal dominant or an autosomal recessive inheritance. It is thought that there may be two separate single gene forms of Klippel–Feil syndrome.

Sometimes antenatal scanning can pick up the spinal abnormalities.

CHARACTERISTICS

The most usual form of Klippel–Feil syndrome is characterized by a **short neck** with folds of skin passing to the shoulders to give a **webbed** appearance. This is due to the fusion of one or more of the cervical or thoracic vertebrae. As a result of this fusion **neck movements** are limited, particularly the side-to-side and rotational movements. Flexion and extension movements are often easily performed. (Occasionally the abnormal fusion of the vertebrae extends to those lower in the spine – the lower thoracic region or even the lumbar region. Under these circumstances movement in these parts of the spine would also be limited.) This limitation of movement is not painful, as it can be with arthritis, for example.

The importance of this abnormality lies in the complications which can occur due to injury of the spinal cord so closely encased in the vertebrae. Symptoms can range from numbness and tingling in arms and fingers to spasticity or paralysis. These symptoms can arise quite spontaneously, or be the result of only a minor fall, stumble or knock. The vertebrae which are actually fused are not the problem; rather it is the adjacent ones which are excessively mobile in an attempt to mobilize the whole spine. It is these mobile vertebrae that move out of position and damage the enclosed spinal cord. These symptoms most frequently occur between ten and 20 years of age, the years of maximum activity.

A **low hair-line** at the back of the neck is also a classical sign of Klippel–Feil syndrome.

This triad of signs – a short, webbed neck, limited neck movements and a low hair-line make up the classical Klippel–Feil syndrome picture.

Other **bony abnormalities** are sometimes seen, and include scoliosis, extra ribs in the cervical region and Sprengel shoulder (one shoulder higher than the other.)

Other more unusual associated abnormalities can include:

- defects in the **urinary system**, such as horseshoe kidneys;
- **eye** problems, such as squint, nystagmus or ptosis;
- **cleft palate**;
- **deafness** of either a sensori-neural, or conductive type;
- **cardiac abnormalities**, particularly ventricular septal defects.

All these associated characteristics occur in only a small proportion of sufferers from Klippel–Feil syndrome and certainly would not occur all together in one individual.

MANAGEMENT IMPLICATIONS

The fusion of the cervical vertebrae with the relative instability of the adjacent vertebrae must always be borne in mind when caring for a child with Klippel–Feil syndrome. Contact sports in which the cervical spine, or indeed any part of the spine, could be damaged must be avoided. Interests in more sedentary activities should be encouraged. If damage to the spinal cord does occur, either spontaneously or as the result of injury, urgent surgical stabilization is necessary.

Other **bony abnormalities**, such as scoliosis or Sprengel's shoulder, may also need surgical intervention to prevent the deformity worsening and/or to further improve mobility.

Any **renal abnormality** giving rise to symptoms – perhaps increased liability to urinary infection, for example – must be investigated and remedied where possible.

Deafness must be remembered as a possibility in children with Klippel–Feil syndrome. Hearing should be checked if there is any suspicion that he/she is not hearing properly, perhaps by a fall-off in school performance, for example.

Squints should be treated early if present to prevent amblyopia occurring.

A **cleft palate**, if present, will also need surgical repair. Subsequent speech therapy may also be needed to ensure correct speech.

THE FUTURE

Children with Klippel–Feil syndrome can look forward to a normal life span, provided there are no serious associated kidney problems. Care must be taken at all times to avoid excessive trauma to the neck. An everyday precaution, for example, should be to ensure that adequate head restraints are fitted to any car in which the child, and later the adult, is travelling.

Careers, too, must be chosen with these potential problems in mind.

SELF-HELP GROUP

Klippel–Feil Syndrome Group
c/o Contact-a-Family
170 Tottenham Court Road
London W1P 0HA
(Tel. 0171 383 3555)

Aims and provisions: support for families with the condition; information sheet available.

Lawrence–Moon–Biedl syndrome

ALTERNATIVE NAME

Lawrence–Moon syndrome.

INCIDENCE

In the past confusion has arisen between this syndrome and Bardet–Biedl syndrome, both of which have many similar features. Both syndromes are characterized by learning disability, visual problems, small genitalia and spasticity.

The true incidence is not known, but it has been reported that Arab populations in Kuwait have a higher incidence than is found elsewhere. Boys and girls seem to be affected equally.

HISTORY

The Lawrence–Moon–Biedl syndrome was first described as long ago as 1866. The Bardet–Biedl syndrome was recognized in 1920, together with the similar features to be found in both syndromes. It is only in recent years that the two syndromes have been classified as two distinct entities.

CAUSATION

The mode of inheritance is autosomal recessive. This syndrome is one in which the signs and symptoms become progressively worse as life continues. Due to this fact, it is thought probable that some enzyme defect – as yet undetected – accounts for the typical features.

Genetic counselling is indicated when a child in the family has been diagnosed as having Lawrence–Moon–Biedl syndrome.

There is no specific antenatal test available at present.

CHARACTERISTICS

There are four main features of the Lawrence–Moon–Biedl syndrome.

Learning disability is invariably present, although to a variable degree, ranging from children who are only mildly affected to those with a severe learning disability. This disability becomes progressively obvious as development proceeds. Routine developmental clinics should pick up the specific areas of delay, which are generally of a wide-ranging global nature.

Visual problems, in the form of retinitis pigmentosa, again becomes apparent as the child matures. Difficulty in seeing in the dark, and eventually complete night-blindness, will be noticed as soon as the child is able to verbalize his/her difficulties in this direction. On ophthalmic examination, the retina is found to be thinned, with excess pigment visible first of all on the periphery of the retina. This pigmentation later extends to affect central vision.

Ataxia becomes noticeable at the time when walking should be becoming stable. This distressing feature gradually progresses until eventual paralysis occurs, with spastic limbs.

Sex organs, obvious in boys, are small and underdeveloped. This is present from birth, but may only be noticeable later in life when lack of further development is obvious.

MANAGEMENT IMPLICATIONS

As the **developmental delay** becomes obvious with serial developmental checks, help in specific areas, such as speech and basic learning skills, can be given.

Later, when schooldays approach, full multidisciplinary assessment will be necessary to determine the most suitable educational facilities for the child with Lawrence–Moon–Biedl syndrome. As time passes and, regrettably, progressive physical disabilities occur, the type of schooling will need to be reviewed. Schooling will, of course, depend very much on what is available locally.

Vision will deteriorate as the child matures. Sight will initially be fairly satisfactory centrally, but the child will have diminished peripheral vision. As the pigmentation process extends into the central area of the retina, even this good central vision will be lost. Unfortunately nothing can be done to halt this progressive loss of vision. This loss of vision will also have to be taken into account when schooling is considered.

Similarly, the **ataxia** first noticed in early childhood will become progressively worse until by early adulthood paralysis is complete with spastic limbs.

THE FUTURE

This is bleak for children with the Lawrence–Moon–Biedl syndrome. Progressive visual loss and gradual onset of spastic paraplegia is the gloomy outlook. Parents and children will need much support and sympathetic help during these years.

SELF-HELP GROUP

Lawrence–Moon–Biedl Parents' Support Group
23 Lodge Causeway
Fishponds
Bristol BS16 3JA
(Tel. 01272 654154)

Aims and provisions: contact point for parents and professionals; advice and information for affected families.

Lennox–Gastaut syndrome

ALTERNATIVE NAME

Malignant epilepsy.

INCIDENCE

As the alternative name to this syndrome implies, the Lennox–Gastaut syndrome is a severe form of childhood epilepsy. The actual incidence of the condition is not known, but it is thought that around 10% of children with epilepsy have this syndrome. Again, it is thought that up to 50% of children who have epileptic seizures which are difficult to treat have this syndrome.

Although certain criteria have been laid down before this particular syndrome can be recognized (see below) many authorities consider that this syndrome should be classed under the general heading of epilepsy. It is, however, useful to consider this syndrome as a specific entity when discussing prognosis and treatment.

Boys and girls are equally affected. The features of this syndrome become apparent between the ages of three and ten years – most usually at four to five years.

There is no antenatal diagnosis possible.

CAUSATION

There are a number of events which may possibly be involved in the aetiology of this syndrome:

- the Lennox–Gastaut syndrome can occur in children with existing brain damage.

- in up to one-quarter of cases, the child will have had infantile spasms ('salaam attacks') in earlier childhood (see West's syndrome). It is thought possible that the Lennox–Gastaut syndrome is a later manifestation of this latter syndrome.
- the child showing the typical epileptic pattern of the Lennox–Gastaut syndrome may also have other neurological conditions, such as a brain tumour, a previous severe head injury, a sub-dural haematoma or a congenital condition such as tuberous sclerosis.
- it is thought that genetic factors could account for a small number of cases – around 3%.

CHARACTERISTICS

There are four features which lead to diagnosis of the Lennox–Gastaut syndrome:

- frequent seizures of types varying from recurrent 'absences' through convulsive fits to non-convulsive 'status epilepticus';
- the electro-encephalogram shows a pattern typical of the condition;
- the seizures are especially difficult to control and are resistant to many of the known anti-convulsant drugs;
- regretfully, most children with this syndrome will have learning disability.

As the fits occur in so many random different ways, it can be difficult to diagnose this syndrome. Children can suffer from the most widely known type of fit where the fall to the ground is followed by twitching movements. This type of fit can occur during sleep which can add to the diagnostic problems. Other children, who show the typical EEG pattern of the Lennox–Gastaut syndrome, can have very frequent attacks (sometimes so frequent as to be almost continuous) of 'absences' with head nodding, eye blinking, lack of facial expression and drooling. Yet others suffer from 'drop' attacks, where there is a sudden unexpected fall to the ground. This latter can occur with or without twitching movements.

In addition to these frequent seizures, the child can develop **behaviour problems**. These can include many autistic features as well as many bizarre mannerisms and can be especially difficult to cope with if they are first manifested in the playgroup or early school situation before a definitive diagnosis has been made.

Intelligence will gradually deteriorate with the continuation of the seizures. The cause of this unhappy fact is not clear. It may be that the continual fits damage brain function, or it may be that both the fits and the learning disability have a common underlying pathological cause.

INVESTIGATIONS

The electro-encephalogram will show the typical pattern associated with this syndrome.

MANAGEMENT IMPLICATIONS

First and foremost, all efforts must be made to control the seizures with **anti-convulsant drugs**. As mentioned before, this can be extremely difficult and may never be wholly successful. It is vital that the child's medication is kept under regular review. Steroids have been tried to control the fits, but have not been entirely successful.

For the child with frequent 'drop' attacks, a well-fitting **protective helmet** is necessary to prevent frequent head injury.

A **ketogenic diet** has been tried for some children with intractable epilepsy, with varying degrees of success. This diet is high in fats and tri-glyserides, and must only be given under dietetic and paediatric control. (Trials of this diet were begun when it was noticed that the seizures tended to improve when the child had a feverish illness. So a diet which mimicked the physiological conditions seen in a feverish illness was tried.)

Operative procedures on the brain for children with repeated 'drop' attacks are currently being evaluated.

Schooling will need to be very specialized to cope with both the frequent seizures and the learning disability. It is also important to realize that the child's physical state, and hence abilities, can vary markedly from day to day. Close liaison between health and education authorities is vital.

Respite care for parents will be necessary to enable the rest of the family to go on holiday free from the full-time care of a disabled member.

THE FUTURE

Children with the Lennox–Gastaut syndrome will need care throughout their lives. With the difficulties experienced in controlling the seizures and with the probable deterioration in intellectual function an independent life will be impossible.

SELF-HELP GROUP

Lennox–Gastaut Support Group
45 Station Road
Biddulph
Stoke-on-Trent
Staffordshire ST8 6BC
(Tel. 01782 513045)

Aims and provisions: information regarding this syndrome; support by letter and telephone for affected families.

LEOPARD syndrome

ALTERNATIVE NAMES

Multiple lentigines syndrome; cardio-cutaneous syndrome.

INCIDENCE

This is a rare condition, the exact incidence of which is not known, but 70 cases have been described in the literature. Both boys and girls can be affected. This syndrome is also regarded as an association of abnormalities specifically affecting different parts of the body, LEOPARD being an acronym for LEntigines (small dark brown spots); Ocular features; Pulmonary stenosis; Abnormalities of genitalia; growth Retardation; and Deafness. The name is also used as a descriptive feature of the vast number of small dark brown spots seen all over the body, reminiscent of the markings of a leopard.

HISTORY

This syndrome was first described in the late 1960s.

CAUSATION

LEOPARD syndrome is inherited as an autosomal dominant characteristic. The degree of expressitivity varies from individual to individual, some family members being more affected than others. Less severely affected parents can have more severely affected children and vice versa (cf neurofibromotosis).

CHARACTERISTICS

Lentigines, small, dark brown spots, are found all over the face and body of the sufferer of LEOPARD syndrome. These can be present at birth, or can appear gradually over the first three or four years of life. By five years of age these marks are abundant almost everywhere, except the mucous membranes inside the mouth and eyelids. Below the knees the marks also appear in less profusion. Unlike freckles they do not increase in number when the child is out in the sun. They are also darker in colour than freckles, and are also always small in size, never being more than 5 mm in diameter. This is the chief characteristic of LEOPARD syndrome. The other characteristics arise in varying degrees and severity in each individual.

Eyes are set widely apart. There is no other specific abnormality associated with the eyes apart from this characteristic, although occasionally squints may be present.

Pulmonary stenosis is often only mild and consists of a narrowing of the pulmonary artery as it arises from the heart. Only around 50% of children with the LEOPARD syndrome have this abnormality. It is rare for problems to occur with this narrowing even if it is present. There may be other conductive problems in the heart to be seen on ECG tracings. But again, it is rare for problems to arise due to this.

Abnormalities in the sex organs include hypospadias, in which the opening of the urethra onto the penis is in an abnormal position. Under these conditions the opening of the urethra is not at the tip of the penis, but lower down on the shaft of this organ.

Growth retardation is often seen in children with LEOPARD syndrome. This is not excessive, but most children will only reach the 25th centile on the standard growth charts at 18 years of age.

Deafness affects around one-quarter of children with this syndrome. This is sensori-neural in type, and can cause speech delay if it is not noted early.

MANAGEMENT IMPLICATIONS

There is nothing that can be done about the typical skin lesions of this syndrome. Teasing may occur at school, particularly if the name of the syndrome is known! But during the summer months many children have a multitude of freckles on their bodies anyway. So at this time of the year the child with the LEOPARD syndrome will be less embarrassed by his/her skin markings.

Squints, if present, should be treated either orthoptically or surgically. This should be done early to avoid amblyopia, where vision can be much reduced in one eye. (A squinting eye will cause some degree of double vision. To compensate for this the brain will block off one image, leaving the child with only one visual image. Unless the squint is corrected within a comparatively short time, vision in one eye will disappear altogether through disuse.)

Heart defects will rarely cause any problem. They are often only found later in life as an unusual finding unless, of course, the association with the skin markings are noted.

Hypospadias will need assessment as to degree and the effect it is having on urine flow. Surgical correction may be needed if the defect is severe. It is wise to get this done before the boy starts school, if it is thought to be necessary. Much distress can be caused to small boys by an unusual flow of urine.

Deafness will need to be diagnosed and assessed early in the child's life. Speech therapy may need to be given during the critical years of speech development (around one to three years of age). Deafness during this important time can easily lead to secondary problems with the acquisition of clear speech.

THE FUTURE

The child with LEOPARD syndrome should experience few difficulties due to his/her genetic inheritance. Deafness may be a factor to be considered in the choice of a career, but apart from this a normal life, and lifespan, can be expected.

SELF-HELP GROUP

There is no specific group for the LEOPARD syndrome, but the following group will provide help and advice for hearing problems:

The Royal National Institute for the Deaf
105 Gower Street
London
WC1E 0AH
(Tel. 0171 387 8033)

Lowe's syndrome

ALTERNATIVE NAME

Oculo-cerebro-renal syndrome.

INCIDENCE

This is a rare syndrome, the exact incidence of which is not known. There are 40 families in the UK recorded as being affected by Lowe's syndrome. The basic cause of the condition is thought to be some metabolic disorder. The exact nature of this problem is not clear at present, but research into various areas are proceeding in a number of centres. Due to the mode of inheritance, only boys are affected.

CAUSATION

Lowe's syndrome is inherited as an X-linked recessive disorder. Women who are 'carriers' of the condition can occasionally be shown to have changes in the lenses of their eyes. These changes rarely cause problems, but can be an indicator that the family has Lowe's syndrome in the genetic inheritance. A family history of present members and ancestors known to have similar characteristics is the best way of estimating the risk to a future pregnancy. There is no antenatal diagnostic test available at present, although the causative gene has now been mapped so that testing may be possible with a positive family history.

CHARACTERISTICS

As the alternative name suggests, Lowe's syndrome affects the eyes, brain and kidneys of babies with this condition.

Cataracts are present in both eyes at birth in all baby boys with the full expression of Lowe's syndrome. These affected lenses are often small in size in addition to the opaqueness of the cataract.

Glaucoma, in which the tension inside the eyeball is high, is also common. It had been suggested that the basic cause for this is the small size of the lens. Due to this the drainage passages of the eyes are effectively blocked.

Squints are also common in babies affected by Lowe's syndrome.

Nystagmus, a flickering movement (usually horizontal) of the eyes can also be present.

As the baby matures the eyes do not grow in proportion to the rest of the face. This results in the eyes having a sunken appearance later in childhood.

All these potential problems mean that most Lowe's children will be blind, or at best, only partially sighted.

Renal problems: at birth, and for a few weeks afterwards, kidney function appears to be normal, but after this time the tubules in the kidneys fail to function adequately. This causes wide-ranging chemical abnormalities due to defective excretion of these substances. This has a number of 'knock-on' effects, resulting in failure of growth, hypotonic muscles and a generalized acidosis. The abnormalities in the kidneys become progressively worse as the child matures. Renal failure is frequently seen in mid-childhood.

Mental abilities vary markedly in the boy with Lowe's syndrome. He may have completely normal mental abilities, or may have some learning disability ranging from only very mild to severe. Routine developmental testing will bring to light the areas in which help is needed.

MANAGEMENT IMPLICATIONS

Eyes: full assessment by an ophthalmologist is necessary to determine the full extent of the visual disability. Glaucoma, cataracts and squints will need to be treated to ensure that as much vision as possible is saved. Magnification and good lighting will allow the boy to use what vision he has to the best advantage. Regular testing of vision should continue for as long as there is any measurable vision.

Renal problems must also receive skilled care. Correction of the acidosis, and the hypophosphataemia which is also a common feature, will increase the quality of life for the child – and his parents. Renal failure must be treated appropriately as and when it arises. Early recognition of renal failure, and subsequent active treatment, can increase lifespan.

Mental abilities must be checked routinely as an on-going measure. All skills, such as walking, speaking and self-help skills should be charted. In this way progress, or lack of it, can be measured over the years. Regrettably, many of the boys with Lowe's syndrome are found to have severe learning disability fairly early on in childhood. (But this is by no means invariable as some boys are able to work and play alongside their peers in spite of their poor vision.) But if learning disability is found to be present, suitable schooling will have to be arranged for the child, either in a special school or in a unit with appropriate facilities.

Behaviour problems can also occur. Frustration, along with a degree of learning disability, is the most likely cause of this difficult behaviour. The help of a clinical psychologist can be valuable under these circumstances.

THE FUTURE

This is not good for the boy with Lowe's syndrome. Many boys die before their tenth birthday, usually from renal failure. Some boys reach adolescence and adulthood. Due to poor vision and possible learning disability only very few boys pursue an independent life.

SELF-HELP GROUP

Lowe's Syndrome Association
29 Gleneagles Drive
Penwortham
Preston
Lancashire PR1 0JT
(Tel. 01772 745070)

Aims and provisions: mutual support; educational and medical information; publicity to increase public awareness of the condition.

Marfan's syndrome

ALTERNATIVE NAMES

Arachnodactyly; Marfanoid hypermobility syndrome.

INCIDENCE

Marfan's syndrome is comparatively common, the condition occurring in at least one in every 10 000 of the population. Both sexes are equally affected.

HISTORY

Several of the signs of Marfan's syndrome are not exclusive to the condition, but are also found amongst the general population. So, it has been determined that to make an accurate and correct diagnosis of Marfan's syndrome, at least three of the specific signs or symptoms should be present. If a first-degree relative, i.e. mother, father, brother or sister, also has Marfan's syndrome, two of the characteristic features only are required to make a positive diagnosis.

CAUSATION

Marfan's syndrome is inherited as an autosomal dominant, but some cases arise sporadically as new mutations. Even if the abnormal gene is present, all the typical characteristics may not be seen in any one individual. For example, only the tall stature may occur, without the other specific signs.

Recently a particular protein is thought to be one of the affected substances producing some of the clinical signs. Similar features to those seen in Marfan's syndrome can occur in another disorder, homocystinuria. Amino acid assay of the urine is needed to distinguish between the two disorders.

CHARACTERISTICS

Skeletal system

Tall stature: all Marfan's syndrome children are tall, being taller than their classmates from an early age. Long slender limbs, which look out of proportion to normal sized trunks make up for this increased height (cf achondroplasia).

Vertebral column abnormalities: there can be a scoliosis (a sideways bend) to the spine in the thoracic region. Also, a kyphosis can occur in this region of the back, giving rise to the appearance of rounded shoulders.

Fingers and toes are also particularly long and slender – often giving rise to the name 'spider fingers'!

Joints are either very mobile or alternatively can be stiff and contracted. The former is the more common, and is especially noticeable in the wrists, elbows and fingers. Dislocation of joints can occur more readily than normal due to the laxity of the joint capsule and the comparative weakness of the muscles surrounding the joint.

Chest: there are frequently deformities of varying types and degrees in this region of the body.

A **high, arched palate** is also a consistent feature.

Eyes

In a high proportion of children with Marfan's syndrome, the lenses of the eye are dislocated, giving rise to poor vision. In addition to this, myopia (short-sight) is common. Detachment of the retina occurs more frequently than in the general population. Squints and/or nystagmus can also occur, but neither is an invariable characteristic.

Cardiovascular system

The **aorta**, the large artery passing oxygenated blood from the heart to the rest of the body, is often dilated in its upper part. This can lead to the development of an aneurysm (a 'blowing out' of the blood vessel) in later life.

The **valves** of the heart can also be affected, the mitral or aortic valves being the ones most commonly affected. The valves are lax and can prolapse, causing problems of inadequate blood flow through the heart.

These cardiac defects are all part of the connective tissue disorder.

Mental abilities

Children with Marfan's syndrome have normal intelligence. Occasionally it has been reported that attention span can be limited and also that verbal performance, on testing, can lag behind comprehension. This is by no means always the case, but there is strong evidence that these types of problems do affect Marfan children more frequently than children in the general population. So it is important that regular checks on school performance are made.

Other features

Subcutaneous tissue can be reduced. This leads to excessive slimness which adds to the 'long, lean look'.

Muscles can be weak, so that Marfan's children are not natural sportsmen and women.

MANAGEMENT IMPLICATIONS

Skeletal system

Scoliosis should be noted early before the deformity becomes marked. Scoliosis, if left untreated, can progress to severe chest deformity with subsequent cardiac and respiratory problems. So, early bracing or operative procedures should be done to reduce the possibility of further problems. Any bracing procedures must, however, be done very carefully as respiratory problems can result. In girls, early puberty has been induced by the giving of appropriate hormones. This both reduces final height, and can also prevent the worsening of the scoliosis during the period of rapid growth seen during puberty.

Joint contractures occur in a minority of children. Physiotherapy, if given early and consistently, can do much to maintain mobility, which can be at risk due to the joint problems.

Eyes

Checking on visual acuity early is vital, so that corrective lenses can be given to counteract the myopia which is so common.

Squints, if present, will need to be corrected, either orthoptically or surgically if amblyopia is to be avoided. This is important, as visual acuity is compromised in children with Marfan's syndrome anyway due to the other eye abnormalities. The dislocated lenses, which of course also reduce vision, should be left in position. In the past lenses have been removed surgically, but it has subsequently been found that this predisposes to retinal detachment.

Cardiovascular system

Beta-blocker drugs, given on a long-term basis, have been found to reduce the rate of dilatation of the aorta. Operative procedures may be necessary to replace the dilated aorta at a later date. Some authorities recommend repair of the dilated aorta when the size of this blood vessel has reached 6 cm, even without symptoms. Surgery may also be necessary on the abnormal valves in the heart. Endocarditis, an infection of the inner layer of cardiac muscle, is a possible complication. Because of this possibility, antibiotics should be given prophylactically before minor operative procedures, such as dental extractions, for example.

Due to the cardiac, visual and skeletal problems which Marfan's children suffer, certain restrictions should be put on their physical activities. For example, body contact sports must be avoided due to the possibility of damage to the eyes, and sports which require the body to be pushed to its physical limits, such as marathon running and weightlifting, must be avoided. The heart, under these circumstances, has a heavy load to bear, and with the possible abnormalities to be found in Marfan's syndrome, such exertion can lead to cardiac failure. Weak muscles and skeletal problems will also, in many cases, exclude many of the more strenuous physical activities.

Mental abilities

Children with Marfan's syndrome will be able to manage intellectually very adequately in mainstream schooling, but in some cases visual problems may be sufficient to need special schooling for partially sighted pupils.

The possibility of a specific attention deficit must also be remembered and appropriate action taken in school to be aware of, and remedy, the problem.

THE FUTURE

Children with Marfan's syndrome may have a reduced life expectancy due to the cardiac problems. Around 40 to 50 years is the usual life span. Complications due to the aortic abnormalities account for 90% of early deaths. As long as sensible precautions are taken not to overload the cardiovascular system, a normal life can be led within the limits of reduced vision. This, of course, will vary from individual to individual. Genetic counselling before a pregnancy is embarked upon is advisable.

SELF-HELP GROUP

Marfan Association
6 Queens Road
Farnborough
Hampshire GU14 6DH
(Tel. 01252 547441)

Aims and provisions: dissemination of information to public and professionals; fostering of research projects.

Moebius syndrome

ALTERNATIVE NAMES

Congenital facial diplegia; Moebius sequence.

INCIDENCE

This is a rare syndrome, but one which nevertheless has important implications for the care of new-born babies. Boys and girls are equally liable
to be affected.

A link between Moebius syndrome and two other similar syndromes,
the fascinatingly named 'Charlie M' syndrome and Poland syndrome, has
been hypothesized. These two latter syndromes have abnormalities in face,
arms, fingers and chest muscles as well as facial problems. It has been
suggested that a failure of development of specific blood vessels at a
critical stage of antenatal life is the basic cause of these abnormalities.
Both Charlie M and Poland syndromes are incredibly rare.

CAUSATION

This is controversial. Most cases are thought to be sporadic and due to a
new mutation but an autosomal dominant inheritance is also thought to
be possible. One family, having the syndrome in three successive generations, had chromosomal abnormalities, but this has not been reported
again. Yet another suggestion as to the aetiology of this syndrome is illness,
drug abuse or accident in the mother during the first three months of
pregnancy. There is no antenatal test available. Moebius syndrome can be
recognized at birth by the lack of facial movement.

CHARACTERISTICS

The main effects of Moebius syndrome are found in the **face.** The baby is born with almost complete lack of movement in his/her face, usually on both sides. Little facial expression is ever seen, and the baby's eyes and mouth remain open for most of the time. Occasionally only the upper part of the face (both sides) is affected. The facial muscles are supplied by specific cranial nerves, arising straight from the brain stem, and studies have been done in relation to these nerves. In a few well-studied cases, the nuclei (the 'power-house' of the nerve) have been seen to be small and under-developed.

In addition to weakness of the facial muscles, there is frequently also weakness in those of the palate and tongue. All these muscles are intimately connected with sucking and swallowing, thereby making feeding difficult in the new-born baby. Occasionally tube feeding may be necessary to ensure that he/she obtains sufficient nutrition for growth.

Aspiration into the lungs of milk, or even only saliva and mucus, is a real threat in these young babies. If this occurs, broncho-pneumonia can be the result.

As the baby matures many of these problems improve, although solid food can become lodged in the cheeks of the older child. This is due to the continuing difficulty he/she will be having with his/her facial muscles.

Eyes must be watched carefully for scratching and possible ulceration of the cornea. This occurs due to the inability of the baby to close his/her eyes fully. Minute particles of dust in the atmosphere can remain on the delicate tissue of the cornea and not be washed away by normal blinking.

Speech: difficulties can be experienced in the proper articulation of words as this skill is obtained. The child's weak facial muscles make it difficult for him/her to move the lips and tongue together to shape and form sounds.

In some babies with Moebius syndrome there may also be abnormalities of the **fingers.** These can either be small and shortened or long and slim.

Chest muscles can also be affected in this syndrome, in some cases being absent altogether.

Talipes is an added finding in 35% of babies with Moebius syndrome. These last three aspects overlap with those seen in Poland syndrome.

MANAGEMENT IMPLICATIONS

Most of the acute problems are encountered during the early months of life, **feeding** in particular being a problem. Tube feeding initially may be necessary to prevent aspiration of milk and also to avoid exhaustion in the young baby. With weak facial muscles he/she will have to work twice as hard to gain the same amount of milk as his/her more robust contempor-aries .

Although the facial muscles will never be normal, the baby and older child will eventually learn to cope adequately with swallowing, although sucking may be a continuing problem. Food lodged in cheeks can cause choking in the toddler whose feeding patterns are not fully established. So throughout childhood, careful watch must be kept at meal times on children with Moebius syndrome.

Any aspiration problems with the potential to lead to **aspiration pneu-monia** must be recognized early and treated energetically.

Early recognition and treatment of **corneal abrasions** is also vital to prevent corneal scarring. Any redness in the baby's eyes, or excessive watering or obvious discomfort should receive immediate attention.

Speech therapy is of great importance to ensure that understandable speech develops in the child with Moebius syndrome. This should be started early, from around 18 months of age. This will ensure that unco-ordinated attempts to pronounce words are reduced to a minimum. Parents will also be able to obtain valuable advice on how best they can help their child with this vital skill.

THE FUTURE

Moebius syndrome will not exclude the child and young adult from many activities. However, lack of facial expression and possible difficulties with articulation may obviously make for problems with a career or leisure activity which calls for appearing before the public.

Once the early years are successfully passed, life and lifespan can be practically normal for Moebius syndrome sufferers.

Genetic counselling should be offered to affected families.

SELF-HELP GROUP

Moebius syndrome contact group
21 Shields Road
Whitley Bay
Tyne and Wear NE25 8UJ
(Tel. 0191 253 2090)

Aims and provisions: support and advice to affected families.

Morquio's syndrome

ALTERNATIVE NAMES

Mucopolysaccharidosis 4; Brailsford syndrome.

INCIDENCE

Morquio's syndrome is one of the mucopolysaccharide abnormalities. The mucopolysaccharides are complex sugars which require a variety of enzymes for their correct metabolism. There is a group of diseases, known as the mucopolysaccharides, each of which has a specific enzyme defect. These effects are far-reaching, affecting many organs and tissues of the body. The main problem is the accumulation of mucopolysaccharides in various organs which gives rise to specific symptoms.

About one in 100 000 live births exhibit Morquio's syndrome, and both sexes are equally affected.

There appear to be two sub-types of Morquio's syndrome, one being milder than the other, but having similar signs and symptoms.

HISTORY

Morquio initially described a family in which both the parents and the grandparents of the affected child were closely related. This gave the clue to the genetic basis of the disease. With the advance of biochemical and genetic knowledge, Morquio's syndrome is now known to be one of the mucopolysaccharide diseases. (See also Hunter's, Hurler's and San Filippo syndromes.)

CAUSATION

Morquio's syndrome is inherited as an autosomal recessive. The complex sugar involved in this particular mucopolysaccharide disease is keratan sulphate. Excessive amounts of this substance are excreted in the urine of many children affected by Morquio's syndrome, but in some children this substance is not found to be present. However, deficiency of the enzyme involved in the metabolism of keratan sulphate can be found by laboratory tests in all sufferers. Antenatal diagnosis can be made by chorionic villus sampling or amniocentesis.

CHARACTERISTICS

Antenatal growth and development proceed normally, and this continues throughout the early months of life. But by around 18 months of age the following characteristics begin to appear.

Growth retardation: weight and height development are seen to slow down from 18 months or so onwards. By the age of five years, no further growth occurs, with final height rarely reaching more than 32 inches (80 cm).

Skeletal changes: the spine and chest become severely deformed, with a marked kyphosis and scoliosis, i.e. the spine being twisted both forwards and sideways. The ribcage is short and broad and the ribs have a flared appearance at the base. The breastbone is very protruding, giving rise to a pigeon-chested appearance. The neck is seen to be shortened, due to failure of proper development of the upper vertebrae. Lack of development of this part of the spine can lead to compression of the spinal cord later in life, giving neurological signs and symptoms in the arms and legs at this time.

Limbs: the arms are relatively long, all joints are lax, the wrists and fingers being particularly affected. Legs are short due to the general lack of growth and knock-knees and flat feet are common.

Teeth, both the first and second set, have abnormal enamel. Due to this lack of protective enamel infection can be rampant and tooth decay is a further, painful problem.

Deafness is common in children with Morquio's syndrome and again is a direct result of the accumulation of the specific complex sugar involved in the disease.

Cardiac defects are to be found in some children. The most usual problem is failure of development of the aorta.

Eyes: clouding of the cornea, a common occurrence in all the mucopolysaccharide diseases, is frequently seen in children with Morquio's syndrome.

The **intelligence** of children with this syndrome develops normally, so they are able to benefit from normal teaching within the constraints only of their physical capabilities.

Secondary sexual characteristics develop normally.

MANAGEMENT IMPLICATIONS

Spinal problems: the abnormalities in the upper cervical vertebrae frequently give rise to compression of the spinal cord. This is due both to the abnormalities in the vertebrae themselves and to the laxity of the ligaments in this part of the body, in common with the lax ligaments around other joints. From this compression weakness in the legs results, together with tingling sensations. Without adequate treatment, paralysis can result. Spinal fusion of the affected vertebrae can prevent, or cure, this problem. Carers of children with Morquio's syndrome should be aware that this complication can occur and be alerted to the possibility by complaints of increasing weakness in the legs and/or increased difficulty in walking. Physiotherapy can be helpful in strengthening leg and arm muscles so that movement is easier. This will also reduce strain on joints with their weak ligaments.

Short stature will create problems with school and work equipment. Specially adapted chairs and tables will help the child with Morquio's syndrome as he/she reaches secondary school age. Stairs and long corridors that need to be traversed during the course of a school day can also pose problems. These factors must all be borne in mind when helping the Morquio child obtain full benefit from the education system.

Clothing can also be difficult due to the unusual body shape. If at all possible, hand-made clothes are most suitable, and this can be an interesting hobby for children – and adults – with the condition.

Work prospects will depend on finding suitable employment for people of such short stature, whilst also bearing in mind other problems such as deafness and possible poor vision.

Hearing must be assessed regularly. Any loss can be helped by fitting hearing aids.

Tooth decay must be treated adequately by regular dental care and by fitting crowns or dentures where necessary.

THE FUTURE

Life expectancy for the child with Morquio's syndrome is reduced by cardiac and neurological complications. These frequently lead to death at an early age, usually in the twenties. This is the situation found in children with the most severe form of Morquio's syndrome. The milder type of Morquio's syndrome has a longer life expectancy.

SELF-HELP GROUP

The Society for Mucopolysaccharide Disease
55 Hill Avenue
Amersham
Buckinghamshire HP6 5BX
(Tel. 01494 434156)

Aims and provisions: support and advice for parents; fund-raising for research and grants; annual parent weekend conference; videos giving help with day-to-day problems.

Nephrotic syndrome

ALTERNATIVE NAME

Finnish type nephrosis (primary category only)

INCIDENCE

There are two broad categories of the nephrotic syndrome – primary and secondary. The primary type includes nephrosis arising as a congenital abnormality, which was mainly described in Finland (hence the other name of Finnish type nephrosis). The exact incidence of this type is not documented, but both sexes are known to be affected, with perhaps a slight preponderance of boys. Other primary types arise with no known predisposing cause. Secondary types of the nephrotic syndrome can be caused by a variety of infections, such as toxoplasmosis, cytomegalovirus and syphilis as well as mercury toxicity and a wide range of other conditions such as Henoch-Scholein purpura and other connective tissue disorders.

The overall incidence of the nephrotic syndrome differs in various parts of the world, but is thought to affect around three to four children in every 100 000 in Caucasian populations. In 1985, a higher incidence was reported amongst the Asian population in Britain – around 12 to 16 children per 100 000 suffering from the disease. No account was given for these higher numbers. Many cases in West Africa arise as a result of a particular form of malaria.

CAUSATION

The congenital type of the nephrotic syndrome is probably inherited as an autosomal recessive disorder.

As already discussed, there is an enormously wide variety of causes for secondary nephrosis. Some cases also arise completely out of the blue, with no predisposing condition apparently being involved.

The basic pathological changes giving rise to the typical characteristics of the disease, occur in the kidneys.

CHARACTERISTICS

Whatever the cause of the nephrosis, similar features occur, due to the pathological changes in the kidneys.

Signs and symptoms of other underlying conditions – infectious, toxic or auto-immune – will, of course, also be seen in each individual child suffering from the disease.

Swelling, in many parts of the body, is often the first noticeable feature. This is frequently especially evident around the child's eyes, causing them to appear as mere slits. Initially this can often be put down to an allergic disorder, but as swelling appears in other parts of the body the true diagnosis becomes evident.

Fluid can be retained in the lungs and abdomen giving rise to **breathlessness** and/or **abdominal pain**.

The child will be **lethargic** with a poor **appetite**, and may also have bouts of mild **diarrhoea**.

Urine output becomes diminished, and the urine that is passed contains much protein.

There is frequently a history of **upper respiratory tract infection** before these symptoms appear, lending credence to the hypothesis that infection in some way plays a part. (The nephrotic syndrome is characterized by relapses of the disease over the years, and a head cold often seems to be the precipitating factor in the onset of one of these relapses.)

The usual age group of children to be affected is between the ages of two and ten years, with the exception of the congenital type of nephrosis, when signs of the disease can appear before the age of three months.

INVESTIGATIONS

Specialized tests on the **urine** will make the diagnosis clear. **Blood tests** will also be necessary to determine any underlying causes for the onset of the symptoms due to the kidney involvement. Similarly, **throat swabs** can give clues as to possible infective causes. **Renal biopsy** is sometimes necessary in children where the diagnosis is unclear.

COMPLICATIONS

Extra infection can be a worrying complication of the nephrotic syndrome. A certain type of streptococcus bacteria is the most common infecting organism. Peritonitis (infection in the abdominal cavity) is probably one of the most usual, and difficult to diagnose, infections. This can also present especially difficult problems if the child is receiving steroids as part of the treatment for the initial disease. Signs and symptoms are frequently altered by these powerful drugs.

Thrombosis (abnormal clotting) in either veins or arteries is also an increased risk for children with the nephrotic syndrome, due to the high levels of fibrinogen and other clotting factors seen in this condition. Signs and symptoms will depend on which part of the body is affected.

MANAGEMENT IMPLICATIONS

As mentioned before, the nephrotic syndrome is one which has remissions and relapses. This long drawn out sequence of events in this chronic disease can be very frustrating and wearing for both parents and child.

During the initial attack parents will need full explanation of:

- the likely course of the disease;
- the effects of treatment;
- danger signs to watch for in the everyday life of their child.

In view of the importance of this educative process, it is preferable that the child should be in hospital initially. Also, it is easier to stabilize the child on a diet and drug regime as an in-patient.

It is important that an adequate **diet** is observed to ensure proper growth. The child with the nephrotic syndrome will probably have a poor appetite anyway, due to the unpleasant features of the disease, so tempting dishes are important. Foods high in salt must be avoided. So the rule 'no added salt at the table' must be enforced with avoidance of salty crisps and other snack foods. (This will not prove popular, but must be insisted upon!) Dietetic help is of great value in the preparation of suitable and attractive meals.

Careful control of **fluid intake** also plays an important part in the control of the disease. The amount of fluid taken each day must be worked out to cause maximum effect without rendering the child dehydrated. Again, parents must be made aware of the need for these restrictions when the child returns home. Occasionally, diuretics (fluid removing drugs) may be needed, but must be used with caution.

Steroids, given orally, are the first-line drugs to be used in this condition. Again, the dosage given must be carefully controlled and monitored. In most children the course of the disease will be altered by these powerful drugs. Repeat urine tests, along with the clinical condition of the child, will determine the efficacy of this drug. As well as benefiting many conditions, steroids also have side effects, some of which are dangerous. Parents should be warned that:

- their child will have an increased appetite, so they will have to be especially careful regarding snack foods;
- energy levels will increase, especially so from the lethargic child they knew before treatment was started;
- it is dangerous to stop taking steroids abruptly. In view of this a 'steroid card' is issued to everyone taking the drugs, This will warn doctors, in cases of accident, that the child needs these drugs;
- they should report to their doctor any close contact the child has had with measles or chickenpox. These two childhood fevers will be very severe – and can prove to be fatal – for people taking steroids unless preventative action is taken. Under these circumstances, passive immunization with immunoglobulin and/or specific antiviral therapy will be needed. Teaching staff at the child's school will also need to be aware of the dangers to the child of contact with these diseases.

Although steroids are beneficial to many children with the nephrotic syndrome, occasionally other drugs are necessary. **Cyclo-phosphamides** are the usual alternative drugs, with other more unusual drugs being held in reserve. Again, careful evaluation of any side effects of this drug will need to be made. Toxic effects on the bone marrow can occur as well as possible later infertility. As with all these useful, but powerful drugs regular checks on responsiveness and side effects are necessary.

After the initial hospitalization to put the child on a stable drug and diet regime it is important that the child's life should return to normal as quickly as possible, with a return to the usual **school** and activities. School teachers must be made aware of the child's condition and drug and diet regime.

THE FUTURE

As mentioned before, the nephrotic syndrome proceeds with periods of relapse and remission. With treatment, the chances of long-term remission are good. Infections should never be treated lightly, however, and special care must be taken at these inevitable times.

SELF-HELP GROUPS

There is no specific self-help group for the nephrotic syndrome, but the two self-help groups below are both concerned with all aspects of kidney disease:

British Kidney Patient Association
Bordon
Hampshire GU35 9JZ
(Tel. 01420 472021)

Aims and provisions: financial support to cover expenses as a result of conditions where necessary; fund-raising.

National Kidney Foundation
6 Stanley Street
Worksop
Nottinghamshire S81 7HX
(Tel. 01909 487795)

Aims and provisions: information and contact; practical help from local groups.

Neurofibromatosis

ALTERNATIVE NAME

Von Recklinghausen's disease.

INCIDENCE

Neurofibromatosis affects around one in every 3000 live births. There are thought to be about 18 000 sufferers in the UK. The severity of the disease is very variable, some people only having mild symptoms, whilst others can be severely restricted. The sexes are affected equally, and there appears to be no predilection for a specific race.

HISTORY

Dr Friedrich Von Recklinghausen first described the condition in the 19th century. He described the main features of neurofibromatosis shown by 90% of sufferers. Later it was found that there are certain variations which Dr Von Recklinghausen did not describe.

CAUSATION

Neurofibromatosis is a genetically inherited condition; the gene is situated on chromosome 17. The condition is inherited as an autosomal dominant, therefore parents have a 50% chance of passing it on to their children.

CHARACTERISTICS

Cafe-au-lait spots: these are coffee-coloured patches of skin anywhere on the body. Cafe-au-lait spots are not uncommon, but people with neurofibromatosis have very many of these patches. The number increases as growth proceeds, as well as the existing marks becoming larger. Any child with six or more cafe-au-lait spots should be examined closely for underlying signs of the disorder. These cafe-au-lait spots cause no problems themselves, apart from cosmetic. The marks are due to an excess of the skin pigment melanin. One further melanin effect which gives a valuable clue in the diagnosis of neurofibromatosis is a marked freckling of the skin in the armpits of children of ten years and over with the condition. Occasionally this is the only sign that the person has the neurofibromatosis gene. (Unfortunately, this does not mean that this person's children will also only have this minor manifestation of the disease. They could be more severely affected.)

Dermal neurofibromatosis: it is this manifestation of the disease that can cause the most problems. These lesions are swellings which appear on the skin in any part of the body. They are not malignant, i.e. they are not cancerous and so do not spread to other parts of the body, but they do tend to increase throughout life. So by the time the sufferer has reached his/her, 'three-score-years-and-ten' there may be very many of these swellings, of all shapes and sizes, present. Usually these swellings do not make their appearance before puberty. Apart from the disfiguring cosmetic effect, dermal neurofibromata can cause problems when they arise in difficult situations, for example, around the waist, neck-line, between buttocks or under shoulder straps. If this occurs they can be removed surgically, but unfortunately this does cause scarring. If they are multiple, they are best left alone. Surgical removal is most applicable to those swellings that are causing discomfort or irritation.

It is on the basis of the above two signs that the diagnosis of neurofibromatosis is made. There are a few other manifestations that can occur, but not necessarily always.

Many people with neurofibromatosis tend to be shorter than the average. There is no underlying defect in the bony tissue to account for this, and the reason is unknown.

Other **skeletal problems** can occur, a scoliosis (a sideways curve in the spine) being one of the most common. This usually occurs during the teenage years – the years of maximum growth. Often no treatment is necessary, as the condition is mild. Swimming is very beneficial for this particular problem, especially in the adolescent years. But if it is more severe, surgery may be required.

Occasionally, the bones of the forearms and legs are thinner than normal.

This can result in a bowing of the legs. Also, fractures can occur more readily in these thinned bones.

Benign tumours, i.e. those that do not spread to other parts of the body, do occur more commonly in neurofibromatosis sufferers than in the general population. These tumours consist of nervous and fibrous tissue as do the dermal neurofibromata. There are three main sites in the body which can be affected:

- The **spine**: tumours can occur in the nerve roots arising from the spinal cord. The signs and symptoms that arise from these will depend on the actual site of the lesion in the spinal cord. Weakness, numbness and possibly pain, will occur in that part of the body supplied by the affected nerves. If the tumour arises in the lower back region, bladder control can also be affected.
- The **ear**: a tumour arising on the eighth cranial nerve (the nerve associated with hearing) will cause gradual loss of hearing. Giddiness may also occur, as can weakness of the facial muscles on the affected side. (A very rare type of neurofibroma, known as a 'central neurofibroma', involves tumours on both auditory nerves. These develop quite independently of each other and can cause bilateral deafness. Sufferers from this rare condition do not usually have cafe-au-lait spots or dermal neurofibromata.)
- The **eye**: the optic nerve can also be the site of a neurofibroma. Signs and symptoms of this will include a developing squint and blurred or double vision.

All these tumours can be removed successfully. Obviously, surgery is easier if the tumours are small. So any complaint of deafness, altered vision or weakness in limbs in a person with neurofibromatosis must be urgently investigated.

Plexiform neurofibromatosis: this type of neurofibroma is exceedingly rare. It consists of complex overgrowths of nervous/fibrous tissue anywhere in the body and can be extensive in size.

Learning difficulties: there is a slightly higher incidence of reading and writing difficulties in children with neurofibromatosis than in the general population.

MANAGEMENT IMPLICATIONS

Dermal neurofibromata: watch must be kept on the development of new swellings, especially in problem sites. Treatment consists of surgical removal of swellings that give rise to irritation or pressure problems. Regular follow-up is ideal.

Deafness, or **visual problems** such as squint or blurred vision, must be investigated early. Accurate diagnosis of the cause, followed by appropriate treatment is essential.

Genetic counselling should be given as the child approaches maturity. Difficult decisions will need to be taken as to whether to have children with the risk that they, too, may be affected.

Blood pressure should be monitored regularly, as there is a higher incidence of a specific tumour of the adrenal gland (phaeochromocytoma) and also narrowing of the renal artery in neurofibromatosis sufferers. Both these conditions will give rise to raised blood pressure.

Non-accidental injury: investigators will need to remember the increased risk of fractures of the long bones in neurofibromatosis sufferers.

Emotional problems associated with neurofibromatosis must not be overlooked. Adolescents are especially concerned regarding skin blemishes, and as the appearance of dermal neurofibromata begins at this time of life, this can be traumatic. Parents will also need support, as their 'guilt' regarding the genetic inheritance of the disease can be very real.

Learning difficulties of a moderate degree can affect neurofibromatosis children to a slightly greater extent than the general population. Falling behind in school work should alert teachers to the possible need for 'statementing' procedures (in the UK) to be undertaken. This will ensure that appropriate schooling is made available for the child. This, in turn, will prevent the development of secondary behaviour problems as a result of frustration and apparent failure in academic subjects. Loss of schooling, on occasions, may have a deleterious effect on some children's education. Surgical removal of dermal neurofibromata may need in-patient treatment for variable lengths of time. Home tuition, or work sent home at these times – especially for children of an age where examinations are an immediate reality – may need to be arranged.

THE FUTURE

This will depend on the presence of complications as well as the actual site of the neurofibromtose growths.

SELF-HELP GROUPS

The Neurofibromotosis Association
82 London Road
Kingston-on-Thames
Surrey KT2 6QJ
(Tel. 0181 547 1636)

Aims and provisions: supports sufferers; promotes awareness of condition; raises funds for medical research; acts as a liasion point for professionals and organizations.

Niemann–Pick disease

ALTERNATIVE NAMES

Sphingomyelinase deficiency; (sea-blue histiocyte disease).

INCIDENCE

There are four types of Niemann–Pick disease – A,B, C and D, which all have an accumulation of sphingomyelin in various tissues of the body as the basic defect. This accumulation is due to a deficiency of the enzyme, sphingomyelinase, which normally breaks down this lipid substance. Type A is the most common, and severe, variant, and occurs mainly in people of Ashkenazi Jewish descent. All types may vary in severity and, therefore, prognosis.

Niemann–Pick disease is a rare disorder; the actual number of cases not being recorded. Both sexes can be equally affected. Antenatal diagnosis is possible for types A and B.

HISTORY

The type D variant is closely allied to type C. It has been traced back to one 17th century French Acadian couple from Nova Scotia. There is a fifth variant known by the splendid name of 'sea-blue histiocyte disease'. This is due to a preponderance of particular cells found in the bone-marrow which are of a foamy or sea-blue appearance. These cells can also be seen in other types of Niemann–Pick disease.

A new classification of the rather confused typing in current use is currently being worked upon.

CAUSATION

Niemann–Pick disease is inherited as an autosomal recessive disorder.

CHARACTERISTICS

Type A Niemann–Pick disease shows up early in life – within the first few months – with an **enlarged abdomen** (cf Gaucher's disease) due to the enlargement of the liver and spleen. The baby will fail to **gain weight** adequately and **developmental progress** will be slow.

The **skin** may also be a yellowish-brown colour with little subcutaneous fat. This latter fact, together with the lack of weight gain, leads to a starved, almost emaciated appearance.

When their eyes are examined with an ophthalmoscope, many of these babies have a **cherry-red spot** on a particular part of the retina.

Regretfully, due to the accumulation of lipid material in various organs of the body, including the lungs, children with this type of Niemann–Pick disease will die within the first three years of life.

Type B Niemann–Pick disease usually becomes apparent early in childhood when the **enlarged abdomen** is noticed (cf Gaucher's disease). (Occasionally it may be early adulthood before milder cases of the condition are noticed.) The swollen abdomen is again due to abnormal deposits of unmetabolized material in the liver and the spleen – the substance in this case being sphingomyelin.

Infiltration of sphingomyelin into the **lungs** can be the presenting feature, with infection and general respiratory difficulties alerting parents to potential problems.

Most children will feel generally **unwell**, and there will be general poor **growth** and health.

In this type of Niemann–Pick disease **developmental delay** is less marked than with type A, and there appears to be no direct central nervous system involvement.

Lifespan can be normal for those people with a later onset of the disease.

Type C Niemann–Pick disease is similar to type D. With this type onset of symptoms can vary widely from being obvious in the very early days of life through to symptoms only becoming apparent in early adulthood.

Again, symptoms of **abdominal swelling** can occur with general symptoms of ill-health and failure to thrive.

Central nervous system symptoms also occur as time passes, with **general development** being progressively delayed and **ataxia** and **fits** being not uncommon findings. Associated with the poor muscular control (accounting for the ataxia), **speech difficulties** can occur.

Regretfully, many children will die in the teenage years.

Type D Niemann–Pick disease, or the Nova Scotia variant, is very similar to type C. Life expectancy is much reduced and 20 years of age is rarely reached.

INVESTIGATIONS

Bone-marrow testing will show the cells specific to the disease. Analysis of samples from the liver and/or spleen will also show the typical storage pattern.

MANAGEMENT IMPLICATIONS

Although there is no specific treatment, at present, for children with this type of abnormal storage disease, parents and carers will need much support in making life as normal as possible for the child with Niemann–Pick disease.

Regular **developmental testing** is necessary to determine the level of the child's abilities. This is especially important in the types of Niemann–Pick disease in which lifespan can be expected to extend beyond the first decade.

In cases of recurrent **lung** infection, seen most frequently in type B, early prescription of antibiotics is vital.

Anti-convulsant drugs may also need to be prescribed if fits are a part of the symptomatology in any individual child.

Removal of the **spleen** may be a necessary procedure in some cases if this organ is grossly – and uncomfortably – overloaded and swollen with excess sphingomyelin.

Schooling will need to be geared to the child's specific difficulties and regular reviews of progress must be made. It must also be remembered that the frequent bouts of illness and possible hospital admissions can further reduce benefits to be gained from education.

THE FUTURE

This can vary greatly from individual to individual depending upon the type of Niemann–Pick disease and its severity. Unfortunately, life expectancy will be good in only a relative minority of cases.

SELF-HELP GROUPS

Niemann–Pick Support Group
Linden bank
Linden Crescent
Hawick
Roxburghshire TD9 9LQ
(Tel. 01450 370356)

Aims and provisions: support for parents; information on the condition and current research.
The following self-help group is the 'umbrella' group which covers the many, and ever-increasing, number of metabolic disease described. The trust represents nearly 2000 families of children affected by some metabolic disease and is growing rapidly.

Research Trust for Metabolic Diseases in Children (RTMDC)
Golden Gates Lodge
Weston Road
Crewe
Cheshire CW1 1XN
(Tel. 01270 250221)

Aims and provisions: information about the various conditions for parents and professionals; support for families in times of crucial life events; newsletter; financial support if necessary.

Noonan's syndrome

INCIDENCE

Noonan's syndrome is thought to occur in as many as between one in every 1000 and one in every 2500 births. The syndrome has a number of features which vary both in individuals and with time, which can make diagnosis difficult. For example, the facial features which at birth are characteristic of Noonan's syndrome, may alter greatly by the time adult life is reached. Also, a sign which is obvious in one individual with the syndrome may be absent in another. It is thought that there may be some adults who have Noonan's syndrome, but who are undiagnosed due to lack of knowledge in the past, so the incidence of the condition may be greater than originally thought. Both sexes can be affected.

HISTORY

Dr Jacqueline Noonan, a paediatric cardiologist, first reported in 1963 the close association of a specific heart defect with short stature and an unusual facial appearance.

At present, there is no specific test, either clinical or biochemical, which can aid diagnosis. So the association of specific physical characteristics are of prime importance in the recognition of Noonan's syndrome.

CAUSATION

Noonan's syndrome is a genetic disorder passed on as an autosomal dominant, but can be, and often is, a sporadic occurrence. At present, there is no antenatal test which can help with diagnosis, but ultra-sonic scanning early in pregnancy may be able to pick up some of the cardiac abnormalities.

Genetic counselling of parents – and siblings when they reach reproductive age – is advisable following the birth of a child with Noonan's syndrome.

It is thought that there may be a close genetic association with Turner's syndrome as many of the characteristics of the two syndromes are similar.

CHARACTERISTICS

There are three main features which characterize Noonan's syndrome. Other features are often also present and can help confirm the diagnosis, but these are variable both in degree and their presence in each individual.

Congenital heart defects are diagnosable at birth, and can be any one or more of the following, though not all these defects will be found in any one child:

- **Pulmonary stenosis**, in which the valve in the pulmonary artery is narrowed or poorly formed. This is the commonest of the heart defects.
- **Atrial septal defect**: this is a defect in the wall between the two upper chambers of the heart.
- **Ventricular septal defect**: this is a similar defect in the wall of the heart between the two ventricles.

Symptoms relating to these cardiac problems will vary according to the type and degree of abnormality. Many children who have been found on routine examination to have a defect will not need treatment and will be able to live a normal life, whilst others will need drugs and/or cardiac surgery for their condition.

Short stature: this is not extreme, as in some of the other syndromes (cf Turner's syndrome or achondroplasia, for example). Children with Noonan's syndrome tend to be at the lower end of the growth range, around the tenth centile. Special charts are currently being prepared for use with children with Noonan's syndrome. These are necessary because 'normal' height gain is not relevant for children with this syndrome whose growth is along different lines. Bodily proportions are correct (cf achondroplasia). Final height – an important factor when discussing the future – can be estimated from serial measurements on appropriate growth charts.

Facial characteristics, as mentioned, are seen in varying degree in each individual with Noonan's syndrome. Also, as the child matures, the distinctive features tend to become less noticeable. Some of the most obvious characteristics are as follows:

- **Eyes** are widely spaced and tend to be large with a downward slant. There is also frequently a ptosis (drooping of the eyelids) which persists throughout life.

- The **neck** tends to be short with a low hair-line and loose folds of skin in the nape of the neck. (This latter characteristic is also reminiscent of Turner's syndrome.)
- **Ears** tend to be low-set and have distinctive lobes which are bent forwards.
- The **nose** frequently has a flattened bridge.

These three main groups of signs – cardiac problems, short stature and specific facial features – make up the major characteristics of Noonan's syndrome. There can be other associated features, such as the following.

Poor muscle tone, which often gives rise to poor sucking in the early months. Mild degrees of clumsiness throughout childhood are also often seen leading to, for example, Noonan children being poor at sports of all kinds, and tending to knock into objects – the typical pattern of the 'clumsy child'.

Undescended testes occur more frequently than usual. Testes can also be of a small size, and infertility may pose problems when the reproductive years are reached.

Intelligence levels are wide ranging, but specific learning difficulties can be encountered, especially when the child is learning to speak. Noonan children tend to mature late and often are seen to prefer to play with children younger than themselves.

It must be stressed that many of these characteristics are to be found also in the general child population. It is only when a number of these occur together that Noonan's syndrome can be confidently diagnosed.

MANAGEMENT IMPLICATIONS

Heart defects diagnosed at birth, or subsequently, must be checked on a regular basis by a paediatric cardiologist. Treatment with drugs and/or cardiac surgery may be necessary in a small number of children.

Feeding difficulties which can occur during the early months of life due to poor muscle tone may need special sympathetic help from staff both in hospital and in the community. With severe feeding problems, which occur rarely, nasogastric feeding may be necessary for a short time in the neo-natal period. Vomiting can also be a feature of Noonan's syndrome. This can be projectile in character, and differential diagnosis from hypertrophic pyloric stenosis is necessary under these circumstances. These feeding difficulties usually resolve themselves within the first few months of life.

Growth must be monitored regularly throughout childhood. Treatment with growth hormone for children who are growing slowly has been tried, but results are yet to be evaluated. Lack of height along with the tendency to immaturity will need to be understood by nursery nurses and later, by teachers. It is all too easy to underestimate a child's potential ability by treating him/her as younger than the chronological age suggests.

Undescended testes: if this problem is present, it will need surgical intervention before school age is reached, both to ensure the best chance of fertility and to reduce the chance of malignant change.

Speech, **vision** and **hearing** problems, which are all marginally more common in children with Noonan's syndrome, will need specific help and treatment. Speech therapy in particular is often indicated for articulation and language delay. Squint and myopia (short-sight) will need appropriate care and correction as will any hearing loss due to secretory otitis medla.

Genetic counselling is advisable for members of the family who have a child diagnosed as having Noonan's syndrome.

THE FUTURE

Children with Noonan's syndrome usually lead absolutely normal lives. In relatively few, cardiac defects need treatment. Severe cases of this aspect of Noonan's syndrome may restrict life expectancy. Shortness of stature is an irritant rather than a severe problem.

SELF-HELP GROUP

Noonan's Syndrome Society
Unit 5
Brindley Business Park
Cannock
Staffordshire WS11 1GD
(Tel. 01922 415500)

Aims and provisions: support and information for families; raises funds for research; publications describing the condition.

Ollier disease

ALTERNATIVE NAMES

Ollier syndrome; enchondromatosis

INCIDENCE

The incidence of Ollier's disease is not exactly known, but the self-help group concerned with the condition is in touch with 50 families in the United Kingdom. Both sexes can be affected.

CAUSATION

At present there is no known genetic inheritance concerned with Ollier's disease, all cases having arisen spontaneously. The basic defect is in the cartilage at the growing ends of the long straight bones of the body, including the bones of the hands as well as the longer arm and leg bones.

There is no known antenatal diagnosis at present.

CHARACTERISTICS

Ollier's disease is characterized by **swellings in the bones** of many parts of the body. These are due to the overgrowth of cartilage in these positions. When the legs are affected there can be **bowing** of the legs as well as some **shortening** of the affected limb. This latter condition is due to the interference of normal bone growth. On the hands bony swellings become obvious as the mass of cartilaginous cells enlarge.

There is no definitive pattern in these bony growths and any of the long bones of the body can be affected in a random fashion. The condition can be confined to one or two bones or can result in generalized deformity in many parts of the body. Fortunately the bones of the head and spine are not involved in this pathological process.

Ollier's disease can be recognized in babyhood, but more frequently diagnosis is made after the age of around two years. At this age the normal rapid growth will bring to light uneven developments in the skeleton. Some children with this condition will experience **pain** at times of maximum growth.

No other system in the body is involved in Ollier's disease. It is important that this condition is clearly distinguished from a similar condition known as **Maffucci syndrome**. In this latter syndrome, there are many haemangiomata (red naevi of varying size) present all over the body. The prognosis for this syndrome is more serious than for Ollier's disease as there is a far greater chance of malignant changes in the bony lesions.

There is a greater tendency to **fracture** of the long bones in Ollier's disease. This occurrence may be the first sign of the presence of the condition.

Short stature can occur if the long bones of the legs are severely affected. As growth slows, so does the development of new cartilaginous lesions. The lesions already present ossify and become hard.

MANAGEMENT IMPLICATIONS

Many children with Ollier's disease will lead perfectly normal lives if only a few bones are affected. It is when growth is inhibited or asymmetric that problems can arise, such as:

- **physical activities** at school, for example, can be more difficult for children with this condition.
- **fractures** can occur with greater readiness than in children with normal bones. (Care must be taken to exclude Ollier's disease in cases of suspected child abuse.)
- **pain**, especially during periods of active growth, can occur. This will need to be treated with analgesic drugs while it persists.
- **schooling** can be in mainstream school as there is no intellectual impairment with this condition. Teachers should be informed of the reason for the sometimes very obvious swellings on their pupil's hands, legs and arms. They should also be warned of possible periods of pain and the possibility of fractures following minimal trauma.

Orthopaedic intervention may be needed in cases of severe deformity. Care must be taken to exclude **malignant change** in any of the bony lesions. This is rare in children with Ollier's syndrome, but can occur, again rarely, in adult life. X-ray examination is necessary if the bony changes become painful and enlarge rapidly.

THE FUTURE

The expected lifespan for a sufferer from Ollier's disease is normal. Malignant changes in the bones are rare, but must always be remembered. Genetic counselling is advisable if pregnancy is considered.

SELF-HELP GROUP

Ollier's Disease Support Group
6 Wyngrave Place
Knotty Green
Beaconsfield
Buckinghamshire HP9 1XX
(Tel. 01494 673301)

Aims and provisions: contact with affected families; information regarding the condition; co-operation with other skeletal dysplasia groups for teaching and research.

Osteogenesis imperfecta

ALTERNATIVE NAMES

Brittle bone disease; Lobstein's syndrome.

INCIDENCE

'Brittle bone disease' is a rare disorder; the number of babies born with the condition being around three to four per 100 000. There appear to be four distinct types of osteogenesis imperfecta and the incidence varies slightly with each type.

Type 1 is the commonest form found in most populations, although type 3 is more frequently found in South Africa amongst the black population. Type 2 is usually so severe that most babies with this manifestation of brittle bone disease are still-born or die in the first few weeks of life. Type 4 is similar to type 1, the main difference being that the 'whites' of the eyes do not show the characteristic blue coloration of type 1.

Children of all races can be affected, and there is no distinction between boys and girls.

Type 1, being the most frequently seen manifestation of this rare condition, will be described.

CAUSATION

Osteogenesis imperfecta is a genetic disease which is inherited as an autosomal dominant. New mutations also account for a a number of babies with the condition. Biochemically there a defect in the production of one of the precursors of collagen, a substance closely involved in skeletal make-up. At present, there is no antenatal test for the disorder.

CHARACTERISTICS

Skeletal changes: all bones, but in particular those of the arms and legs, are especially fragile and prone to fractures after a minimal amount of injury. Toddlers, who fall frequently as a natural part of learning to walk, are especially prone to such fractures. Most children with brittle bone disease will have had at least one fracture before they reach five years of age.

Spinal deformities can occur, both kyphosis and scoliosis, later in life, but this rarely occurs during childhood. In adults this can result in a loss of height.

Eyes: children with type 1 osteogenesis imperfecta have a marked blue colour to the sclera (the white part) of their eyes. This unusual coloration persists throughout life and is a consistent aid to diagnosis of type 1 osteogenesis imperfecta. People with type 4 often have blue sclera at birth, but this gradually fades, until by the time adulthood is reached, eyes look completely normal. Vision is not affected by this manifestation.

Teeth: type 1 is further divided into two distinct sub-groups, one group having specific abnormalities of the teeth. These children have teeth which are a yellowish-brown colour. Teeth are of normal size and shape, but can be easily cracked or broken and must be watched for decay due to the excessive wear seen.

Hearing can be impaired in children with osteogenesis imperfecta. A conductive type of hearing loss is most usual and is due to deformity in the small bones (ossicles) in the middle ear. Sensory hearing loss can also occur in addition to the conductive loss, high frequency tones being most frequently lost.

Blood vessels are also often excessively fragile, so that in addition to frequent fracture on minimal injury, bruising also occurs relatively easily.

MANAGEMENT IMPLICATIONS

Skeletal system: the peak ages for fractures are between two and three years, and again between ten and 15 years of age. These two peaks coincide with the greatest activity periods in the growing child's life. When fractures occur they must be appropriately treated, making sure that the long bones are carefully realigned so that permanent disability does not result. Physiotherapy is often needed after a fracture has healed so that resultant deformity is minimized. Orthopaedic advice on the possibility of procedures to stabilize limbs which have been subjected to repeated fractures is very worthwhile. Rods positioned inside long bones may be considered if fractures are very frequent. Protective splinting of the long bones may be necessary.

It is of vital importance in possible cases of child abuse that the diagnosis of osteogenesis imperfecta is known, both from the point of view of easily fractured limbs and excessive bruising following minimal trauma.

Teeth must receive on-going and adequate dental care. Advanced dental techniques can change the yellow colour of some children's teeth to a more attractive colour.

Hearing must be assessed at regular intervals and hearing aids supplied if necessary.

Schooling: mainstream schooling is the norm for children with brittle bone disease, except for those children who are very severely affected. Teachers must be informed of their pupil's condition, so that they can act appropriately and quickly should any injury be sustained during school hours. Body contact sports should be avoided due to the risk of fractures on minimal injury.

It can be difficult to strike a balance between protecting the child from injury and allowing him/her to lead a normal life. As children with osteogenesis imperfecta mature, they will learn for themselves what activities are best avoided.

Occupational therapy for severely affected children can give insight into suitable and practical activities.

Trials with **calcitonin** and **fluoride** are currently being undertaken in an endeavour to reduce the number of fractures suffered by children with osteogenesis imperfecta.

Counselling in the adolescent years is of importance so that the young person has an understanding of his/her genetic condition, and the care that he/she should take in the future.

THE FUTURE

A normal lifespan can be expected in the vast majority of people with osteogenesis imperfecta, often with very few problems due to their inherited condition.

Careers with minimal physical contact which could result in fractures should be chosen.

Pregnancy in women who are more severely affected can pose problems. The hormonal changes occurring at this time increase laxity of ligaments and so predispose to fractures – again on minimal trauma. Caesarian section is often considered a wise mode of delivery.

SELF-HELP GROUP

Brittle Bone Society
112 City Road
Dundee DD2 2PW
(Tel. 01382 817771)

Aims and provisions: information on sources of medical and genetic advice; advice and help for families; supports research and raises funds.

Patau Syndrome

ALTERNATIVE NAMES

Trisomy D; Trisomy 13--15 syndrome.

INCIDENCE

The incidence of Patau's syndrome is reported as being between one in 6000 to 8000 births.

There is a slightly higher preponderance of boys being born with this syndrome. Due to the multiple, and severe, malformations associated with this condition, between 80% and 90% of the babies born alive with this syndrome die within the first few months of life. Regretfully, those that do survive are severely disabled.

Patau's syndrome has been reported from all over the world.

Chorionic villus sampling between nine and 12 weeks of pregnancy and/ or amniocentesis at 16 weeks of pregnancy can detect this syndrome antenatally. Ultra-sonic scanning can also detect the decreased size of the head in a baby with Patau's syndrome.

There is some evidence to suggest that older mothers (over 35 years old) are more likely to give birth to a child with this syndrome. Paternal age does not appear to have any effect.

HISTORY

This syndrome was first described and classified by Patau in 1960. In 1984, further studies into the genetics of the condition were undertaken in an European study.

CAUSATION

Patau's syndrome is a chromosomal disorder in which, as the alternative name implies, there are three chromosomes in the 13 position (cf Down's syndrome, or trisomy 21). So, as with both Down's and Edward's syndrome, for example, the total chromosome count is 47 instead of the normal 46.

Occasionally a 'mosaic' trisomy 13 can occur. Under these circumstances, not all the baby's cells have the abnormal 47 chromosomes, but contain cells with the normal complement of 46 chromosomes. Boys or girls with this genetic make-up will be less severely affected, and probably mainly account for those children who survive infancy.

CHARACTERISTICS

These are multiple and severe. Only the most severely affected babies will show all the abnormalities, but all babies with Patau's syndrome have **learning disability**, and have varying degrees of **muscular abnormalities**. All boys also have **undescended testes**. These findings alone do not, of course, lead to the diagnosis of Patau's syndrome, but the added problems which can occur are:

- **microcephaly** is present in a high proportion of cases and can be detected antenatally by ultra-sound;
- **cleft palate and/or lip** can also frequently occur;
- extra **fingers** may also be an obvious feature, as is a **single palmar crease**.

These three features are the ones most commonly associated with this syndrome, but the following also occur:

- the baby's **eyes** can also be small, together with a small **lower jaw**.
- the baby's **neck** can be short, with folds of extra surplus skin at the nape.
- defects in the **bones of the skull** may be present. (This feature is rarely found in other chromosomal disorders, and so can be of assistance in the diagnosis of Patau's syndrome before the chromosomal analysis has been reported.)
- **heart defects** of several different types are a frequent feature, as are **renal abnormalities**. These severe, and often fatal, defects are frequently only discovered at post-mortem examination.

A number of other abnormalities can also occur, such as defects in the spine, abdomen and sex organs. The severity and site of these various features varies from baby to baby with this syndrome.

INVESTIGATIONS

To confirm the clinical diagnosis of Patau's syndrome, a chromosomal analysis of the baby's cells must be done. Further investigations into possible heart and renal defects will need to be done as, and when, problems relating to these systems present themselves in the early, difficult days of life.

MANAGEMENT IMPLICATIONS

In the very early days of life, **feeding** can be a problem. This is due both to the poor muscle tone, and to the smallness of the lower jaw found in many babies. Again, if a cleft palate and/or lip is present, feeding problems are worsened.

If the baby survives the early days of life, routine **developmental checks** will need to be done to determine the extent of the learning disability. This is usually severe.

Heart and **renal** defects will need medical intervention as and when they become apparent.

The **cleft palate and/or lip**, too, will need surgical attention as soon as the baby's general condition is stable enough to withstand the necessary treatment.

Parents will need much **support**, physical help and encouragement to cope with their child's many and severe disabilities. Due to the expected short lifespan of the majority of children with this syndrome, preparation for the baby's death must also be a factor in the forefront of the minds of the people caring for the family.

Bereavement counselling must also not be forgotten following the death of the child.

Genetic counselling is also advisable before a further pregnancy, as some cases do arise from a specific translocation.

THE FUTURE

This is bleak for babies born with Patau's syndrome. 95% of babies die by the age of three years and survivors are severely disabled, both mentally and physically.

SELF-HELP GROUP

SOFT UK
Tudor Lodge
Redwood
Ross-on-Wye
Herefordshire HR9 5UD
(Tel. 01989 67480)

Aims and provisions: support, advice and information for affected families; leaflets regarding the syndrome and bereavement support.

Phenylketonuria

ALTERNATIVE NAMES

Folling disease; hyper-phenylalaninaemia; phenylalanine hydroxylase deficiency.

INCIDENCE

The incidence of phenylketonuria is between one in 10 000 and one in 15 000 live births. This condition is found more frequently in Caucasian populations and rarely in black and Ashkenazi Jewish people. Typically, people with phenylketonuria are fair-haired and blue-eyed, although there may be a few exceptions to these features. Both sexes are equally affected by the disease.

There is no routine antenatal diagnosis in current use, but new techniques are being researched for this purpose and for the detection of carriers of the condition. A test is performed routinely on all new-born babies which detects the abnormality at a very early stage.

CAUSATION

Phenylketonuria is caused by the deficiency of a certain vital enzyme (phenylalanine hydroxylase – PAH) which is necessary for the conversion of phenylalanine into tyrosine. As a result of this defect there is a build-up of phenylalanine (which is an essential amino acid) in the blood. It is the excess of this substance that gives rise to the signs and symptoms of this disease.

Phenylketonuria is inherited in an autosomal recessive manner.

CHARACTERISTICS

The enzyme block to the normal metabolism of phenylalanine causes this amino-acid to build up in the tissues of the body with long-lasting and severe effects if it is not controlled by an appropriate diet. A certain amount of phenylalanine is necessary for proper growth, so the diet must be very carefully controlled during the growing years.

If the condition is not diagnosed at birth, the following effects will occur over the weeks and months after birth:

- **Learning disability**, of a moderate to a severe degree, will be the inevitable result of untreated phenylketonuria;
- in the early days of life, severe **vomiting**, and occasionally **convulsions** can occur;
- the baby's **skin** can be dry with a noticeable eczematous rash;
- it has been said that children with untreated phenylketonuria have a 'mousey' smell. This is due to phenylacetic acid (which is present in excess due to the lack of the appropriate metabolic enzyme) excreted in the sweat and the urine;
- expected lifespan may be shortened.

It must be emphasized that the above characteristics only occur when this condition is untreated. With the appropriate dietary care, the outlook for intelligence and lifespan is excellent.

MANAGEMENT IMPLICATIONS

Of prime importance, of course, is the initial **blood test** done within the first few days of life, to detect the condition. Of equal importance in the prevention of learning disability is the early commencement of an appropriate **diet**. This must definitely begin before the baby is one month old.

There is an intermediate form of this condition – known as hyper-phenylalaninaemia – in which the levels of phenylalanine are raised, but not dangerously so. It is thought that this is a less severe expression of phenylketonuria, with perhaps only a relative lack of the appropriate enzyme dealing with the metabolism of this amino acid.

Alternatively, the raised phenylalanine levels may occur transitorily during the first three months of life. A possible explanation of this feature is a delayed maturation of this specific enzyme system. Skilled analysis and follow-up is needed to differentiate between these connected conditions.

The **diet** for children with phenylketonuria is not especially palatable, but with advice from a dietitian, children will accept it. In babyhood days, specially prepared infant formula milks are necessary. But as a certain amount of phenylalanine is vital for growth, this amino acid must not be omitted altogether from the diet. It is given in measured amounts in the diet, with frequent checks on blood levels. Foods with a low phenylalanine level (flour, pasta, biscuits etc.) can be obtained on prescription. A strict diet is usually recommended until the child is at least ten years old. Some relaxation of the diet after this is possible, but blood levels of phenylalanine must still be checked frequently.

Schooling will offer no problem on the intellectual level, but school staff must be aware of the dietary restrictions so vital to the health and well-being of the child with phenylketonuria.

Adolescence can be an especially difficult time when rebellion against the restrictive diet can, understandably, occur. Support and sympathy from dietitians and other carers is necessary during these formative years.

THE FUTURE

The outlook for children with phenylketonuria is excellent both for lifespan and intellectual ability if the diet is adhered to.

Special care will need to be taken during pregnancy. Babies born to mothers with phenylketonuria stand a greater risk of brain damage due to their mother's high phenylalanine levels. This damage can occur during the very early days of pregnancy. Specialist advice should, therefore, be taken well before pregnancy is embarked upon, so that diet can be adjusted to fully stabilize the amount of phenylalanine in the mother's blood.

SELF-HELP GROUPS

National Society for Phenylketonuria (UK) Ltd
7 Southfield Close
Willen
Milton Keynes
Buckinghamshire MK15 9LL
(Tel. 01908 691653)

Aims and provisions: support for families and individuals; advice and information on the condition and dietary regime; catering workshops; holiday weekends; booklets and information leaflets.

Research Trust for Metabolic Diseases in Children (RTMDC)
Golden Gates Lodge
Weston Road
Crewe
Cheshire CW1 1XN
(Tel. 01270 250221)

Aims and provisions: concerned with all types of metabolic disease in children; support and advice for parents and families; leaflets and newsletter available.

Pierre–Robin syndrome

ALTERNATIVE NAMES

Robin anomaly; Pierre–Robin sequence.

INCIDENCE

This is a rare condition, but one which can cause severe problems in infancy. It can exist on its own, or as part of a wider group of rare syndromes all of which have the Pierre–Robin anomaly in addition to other features. Classification of these other syndromes is unclear at present. It is presumed that both boys and girls are affected equally, apart from, of course, the X-linked variety.

CAUSATION

The inheritance pattern of the Pierre–Robin syndrome is not exactly known. There is a possibility that the condition may be inherited as an autosomal recessive. There have also been suggestions that there may be an X-linked variant which has the additional problems of heart abnormalities and club-foot.

There is no antenatal diagnosis possible, although the cleft palate or the small jaw may be seen on ultra-sonic scanning.

CHARACTERISTICS

The features of the Pierre–Robin syndrome are confined to the lower part of the face and mouth. The initial abnormality from which all the other features follow (hence the term 'sequence') is a very **under-developed lower jaw**.

During the process of development, the baby's **palate** frequently has a rounded cleft in its length.

Following on from the initial defect, the baby can have severe **breathing problems** at birth. The small lower jaw causes the tongue to be positioned further back than is usual. As a result of these unusual anatomical features the baby's tongue will be prone to fall back into his/her throat, thereby effectively obstructing breathing (cf Treacher Collins syndrome, but here the abnormality is not as severe as in the Pierre–Robin syndrome.)

Swallowing difficulties, again due to the positioning of the tongue, can cause problems with feeding in the early days.

Fortunately, once the difficulties of breathing and feeding in the early days of life are over, the baby's lower jaw will develop into a normal size in relation to the rest of his/her face. This 'catch-up' growth is especially marked during the first two years of life.

Later on in childhood there may be **dental problems** with overcrowding and irregular teeth in the lower jaw.

Very rarely, there may be some mild degree of **learning disability** due to lack of oxygen in the first few weeks of life when breathing difficulties are at their worst.

The Pierre–Robin syndrome (or sequence) is an interesting example of how one, comparatively mild, abnormality can have a number of 'knock-on' effects which have far-reaching influences.

MANAGEMENT IMPLICATIONS

Breathing difficulties will need intensive care facilities for the first few weeks of life. It is advisable that all new-born babies with the Pierre–Robin syndrome should be nursed in a partially prone position. (The completely prone position should be avoided due to the possible link with the sudden infant death syndrome. In the special care nursery, babies are monitored continually and immediate action can be taken should any problems arise.) This way of lying will allow the baby's tongue to fall forward, rather than backwards into his/her throat, and so avoids obstruction to breathing. Intubation facilities should always be immediately available in the new-born period for babies with the Pierre–Robin syndrome.

Feeding difficulties will also need special care in the early days. Simple measures such as feeding the baby in an upright position may be all that is necessary to ensure adequate nutrition.

If a **cleft palate** is also present, as is often the case, this will again complicate the feeding of the baby. A modified teat and/or a temporary dental plate can help with this initially. The cleft palate will need surgery to close the gap and ensure easier feeding, breathing and speech. This is often delayed until around three or four years of age to allow maximum possible growth of the palate towards the mid-line. Once the early problems are over the baby with the Pierre–Robin syndrome will develop along completely normal lines.

A few extra problems may arise later in childhood, again all arising from the small lower jaw.

Speech therapy may be necessary in the pre-school years to ensure clear speech following the repair of the cleft palate.

Dental care must be given throughout the early years, until all the second teeth have erupted satisfactorily. Orthodontic treatment may be needed to straighten crooked teeth and to ensure a correct 'bite'.

In very rare cases, special educational facilities will be needed for reduced **intellectual ability**. This is possible if the breathing difficulties have been very severe in infancy, but is by no means inevitable. The vast majority of children with the Pierre–Robin syndrome will be of the same average abilities and physical development as their peers during the school years.

THE FUTURE

Most children with the Pierre–Robin syndrome will grow into adults with the same range of abilities and aptitudes as everyone else. The difficulties in the early days of life will only very rarely have any long-lasting effects.

Genetic counselling is advisable before a pregnancy is embarked upon.

SELF-HELP GROUPS

Pierre–Robin Syndrome Contact Group
28a Fairthorn Road
London SE7 7RL
(Tel. 0181 853 1811)

Aims and provisions: support and information.
Additional advice and help can be obtained from:

Cleft Lip and Palate Association (CLAPA)
1 Eastwood Gardens
Kenton
Newcastle-on-Tyne NE3 3DQ
(Tel. 0191 285 9396)

Prader–Willi syndrome

ALTERNATIVE NAME

Prader–Labhart–Willi syndrome.

INCIDENCE

The precise incidence of the Prader–Willi Syndrome is not known, but is thought to be around one in every 15 000 live births. It is a rare disorder, affecting both sexes equally. There are probably a number of older people who have the Prader–Willi syndrome, but who are undiagnosed due to the lack of knowledge in the past regarding the characteristic features of the condition.

HISTORY

The characteristics of Prader–Willi syndrome were documented by three doctors – Prader, Willi and Labhart in 1956. In 1887, Dr Langdon Down (who also described Down's syndrome) described the syndrome, which he termed 'polysardia'.

CAUSATION

The mode of inheritance of the Prader–Willi syndrome is uncertain. About 50% of sufferers have been shown to have a small deletion on the long arm of chromosome 15, whilst other sufferers appear to have a normal chromosome pattern. (There is a connection with Angelman's syndrome ('happy puppet' syndrome) in which there is also, in a percentage of cases, a deletion or rearrangement on the long arm of chromosome 15. It appears that the syndrome that occurs is dependent upon the parent from which the abnormality arises. Prader–Willi syndrome appears to be derived from the father.)

At present, it is not possible to diagnose the condition antenatally.

CHARACTERISTICS

Hypotonia is commonly seen at birth in babies with Prader–Willi syndrome. This gradually improves over the months and years. The birth of babies with this syndrome is often a breech birth, which possibly has something to do with the hypotonia of the baby. Prader–Willi children and adults tend to have difficulties with co-ordination and balance throughout life. This is a direct result of the relative muscle weakness.

Sucking proves a problem due to poor muscle tone, so that feeding difficulties frequently occur during the first months of life. As a result of these problems, the baby can fail to thrive adequately during the first year of life. Other reasons for failure to thrive must also, of course, be checked out.

An **insatiable appetite**, in contradistinction from the early failure to thrive, makes its appearance between the ages of two and four years. This develops into an obsessive eating pattern and unless controlled, can result in gross overweight. The onset of this hearty appetite may be one of the first clues pointing to the diagnosis of Prader–Willi Syndrome. This trait is thought to be due to some abnormality in the specific part of the brain concerned with appetite control. The obesity which often ensues is particularly hard to treat, and behaviour problems can result from attempts to control food intake.

Short stature, with small hands and feet, are common features of the Prader–Willi syndrome. This reduction in size can be seen on scanning antenatally.

Sexual development is limited, particularly in boys with Prader–Willi syndrome. The penis and scrotum are small and underdeveloped. No Prader–Willi man or woman has been known to have children.

Learning disability of a moderate degree is the general rule, although 10% of Prader–Willi children have a normal intelligence. Children with Prader–Willi syndrome are usually out-going and affectionate, but can have outbursts of rage or temper tantrums, in particular when related to eating. These outbursts are short-lived, but can be difficult to control. The best method is to try to manipulate known situations which provoke outbursts. Moods can swing in the opposite direction – to those of exuberant joy – which can be almost as difficult to contain. Again, situation manipulation is the best method to employ to control this problem.

Occasionally **seizures** can occur, and EEG tracings can be abnormal. This is not a common feature, but one which must always be remembered.

MANAGEMENT IMPLICATIONS

Feeding difficulties during the first year of life will need expert help. Breast-feeding for the first few months is to be encouraged if at all possible. Small, frequent feeds, whether of breast or bottle milk will improve weight gain, and ensure that the small, hypotonic baby with Prader–Willi syndrome does not tire.

Other more usual causes of failure to thrive must be excluded, and remedied if found to be present.

The **insatiable appetite** when it appears around the toddler years, can cause great problems. After the feeding problems experienced earlier, parents will be only too delighted that their child is eating well! But as excessive weight is seen to be becoming a problem, a strict dietary regime will be more readily accepted. It is wise to involve professional dietetic advice to ensure that adequate nutrients are taken for growth and development whilst keeping excess weight gain under control. This aspect of the condition can be one of the most difficult to control, especially in the younger age group.

Learning disability, if present, is generally only moderate, although in some cases it can be severe; IQs can range from 20 to 80. Special schooling will be necessary under these circumstances. A regular, sheltered lifestyle with maximum encouragement and understanding should be the aim in the care of Prader–Willi children. As few children will be able to lead an independent life, it is important that appropriate skills training is given from as early an age as possible.

Difficulties with **co-ordination and balance** will need to be considered during schooling and training. The help of a physiotherapist is valuable for maximizing muscle strength and use.

Scoliosis can be a problem in adolescence, unless muscle tone is strengthened. This may need orthopaedic treatment.

Severe behavioural problems: the moods of children with the Prader–Willi syndrome can be very unpredictable. At one moment they can be 'all sweetness and light' and within a few seconds can deteriorate into an angry outburst. These violent temper tantrums can often be triggered off by the constraints necessary to curb appetite – food is of great importance to the Prader–Willi child. If at all possible, confrontational situations should be avoided over this issue. Giving in to requests for extra food can be all too easy under these circumstances, but patterns of bad behaviour can become an established routine leading to yet more dangerous weight gain in the young person with the Prader–Willi syndrome.

Testosterone may be helpful in increasing the size of the penis and scrotum. This does not increase fertility, but can have a beneficial effect on the behavioural problems, as the boy will not be so aware of his physical differences from his peers.

THE FUTURE

Insulin-dependent diabetes is one of the more serious problems that may occur during the adult years. The incidence of this is higher in Prader–Willi sufferers than in the general population. Regular checks on blood/urine glucose levels should be done and any symptoms of excessive thirst, frequent passage of urine or untoward loss of weight investigated urgently.

Problems of **obesity** are high on the risk factor list. Intercurrent respiratory infections can be dangerous for a very overweight Prader–Willi child.

A fully independent life is not usually possible for Prader–Willi sufferers, but work in a sheltered environment can be undertaken.

SELF-HELP GROUP

Prader–Willi Syndrome Association (UK)
2 Wheatsheaf Close
Horsell
Woking
Surrey GU21 4BP
(Tel. 01483 724784)

Aims and provisions: help for parents and carers; education about Prader–Willi syndrome; help for research.

Primary ciliary dyskinaesia

ALTERNATIVE NAMES

Immotile cilia syndrome; Kartagener's syndrome.

INCIDENCE

There are no exact figures for the number of people affected by this syndrome, but it is thought that as many as one child in every 4000 could be affected. Both boys and girls can suffer from primary ciliary dyskinaesia.

HISTORY

In 1933, Dr Kartagener noticed the relationship between frequent chest and sinus infections and certain specific abnormalities of internal organs. This latter abnormality was the switching of position of some organs to the opposite side of the body. This could include the heart; this organ, under these circumstances, being situated on the right side of the chest.

In 1970, the basic problem causing the recurrent sinus and chest infections was found to be an abnormality in the cilia in certain parts of the body. (Cilia are the minute hairs to be found primarily in all parts of the respiratory tract, as well as in other parts of the body generally. Their function is to sweep secretions up and out of the respiratory tract. This is done by the cilia beating gently backwards and forwards.) In this syndrome the cilia are comparatively immobile. This effectively prevents mucus being removed from the respiratory tract. The static mucus then readily becomes infected, giving rise to the well-known symptoms of upper and lower respiratory tract infections.

Dr Kartagener's original findings of the 'situs invertus' (internal organs on the incorrect side of the body) has been found to occur in only some sufferers from primary ciliary dyskinaesia.

CAUSATION

This condition has recently been found to have an autosomal recessive inheritance. There is no diagnostic antenatal test available as yet.

CHARACTERISTICS

Commonly, babies with this syndrome will have some breathing problems at birth, due to difficulties in moving their normal secretions. However, this quickly improves with appropriate neonatal care. Often there are few indications that the child has any specific condition until the early toddler years, although the young baby is often noticed to have thick secretions constantly running from his/her nose. He/she may also suffer from a seemingly permanently blocked nose, which can cause problems with feeding.

During the toddler years, the child will be found to suffer from **frequent upper and lower respiratory tract infections**. Many children do, of course, suffer from frequent coughs and colds at this time of their lives. The child with primary ciliary dyskinaesia, however, will have an almost perpetually running nose, with thick mucus a constant problem. He/she will also have a constant loose cough. The upper respiratory tract infections will frequently extend down into the lungs, with the risk of resultant pneumonia.

Ear infections associated with these bouts of respiratory infection are also common. The thick mucus retained in the middle ear following these infections can also lead to a conductive deafness.

Sinusitis is also often associated with infections, causing headaches and pain in the cheek regions.

Lack of a sense of **smell** is also a common associated problem. As well as missing out on a good deal of pleasure, the person lacking a normal sense of smell may not be alerted to the potential dangers of, for example, leaking gas and bad food.

Bronchiectasis can be the end result of the frequent lung infections. In this condition, the walls of the alveoli of the lungs are destroyed. This effectively reduces the oxygen-exchanging capability of the lungs, and also allows extra excess mucus to accumulate. These lung changes will only occur after a number of years of repeated infection.

Situs invertus is commonly present in children with this syndrome, but does not inevitably occur. The organs involved can vary; for example, only the heart (dextro-cardia – the heart on the right) being involved in some children. Other abdominal organs can also be reversed. Few symptoms need result from these anomalies, but occasionally added heart defects can also be present.

Symptoms of this condition vary, ranging from severe lung problems to only mild recurring chest infections, and the above anomalies may not be linked together for a number of years. But when it is realized that they may be connected, it is possible to test the mobility of the cilia by electron microscopy. A sample of cilia can be obtained by a nasal scraping. This test is expensive and requires skilled interpretation.

Infertility in men is a further problem associated with primary cilary dyskinaesia. The tail of the sperm has an almost identical structure to that of the cilia in other parts of the body. For normal fertilization to occur, this tail needs to be active. In primary ciliary dyskinaesia, this activity is much reduced. This results in the sperm being unable to move sufficiently for fertilization to take place.

MANAGEMENT IMPLICATIONS

Antibiotic treatment, when necessary for severe respiratory tract infections, should be continued for an adequate length of time with maximal doses. Due to the thick secretions found in primary ciliary dyskinaesia, penetration by the antibiotics can be difficult.

Physiotherapy is valuable for the child who is severely affected and unable to cough up his/her sticky secretions. Postural drainage, two or three times a day, will help to prevent build-up of mucus and reduce infection to a minimum. This is especially important in young children, so that later bronchiectasis can be avoided. By the age of nine to ten years children can themselves learn techniques to clear their chests effectively.

Physical activities should be encouraged in children with this syndrome, provided that there is no other medical reason for avoidance of physical activity, such as a heart defect. Outdoor games and similar active pursuits are especially valuable.

Hearing should be checked regularly in all children who have associated frequent attacks of otitis media. If this occurs during the active time of speech development – between one and three years of age – there may be delay in acquisition of this skill. Following treatment of the hearing problem, speech therapy may be necessary under these conditions.

Myringotomy to drain excess fluid from the middle ear may also be necessary. Some authorities advocate the insertion of ventilation tubes ('grommets') to promote drainage of this fluid.

Heart defects, if present, will need appropriate treatment.

THE FUTURE

This will depend on the severity of the ciliary abnormality. Some people will only be mildly irritated by their frequent nasal and sinus infections. Others will be frequently incapacitated by severe lung infections and the effects of bronchiectasis. Due to these lung problems, smoking is inadvisable. The effects of the nicotine will inhibit the action of the cilia in the lungs even further.

Lack of a sense of smell and a mild hearing loss may pass unnoticed unless specifically asked about and/or tested.

Some men will be infertile due to this syndrome.

Life expectancy is not reduced, unless there are associated heart abnormalities, or the bronchiectasis is very severe.

SELF-HELP GROUP

Primary Ciliary Dyskinaesia (PCD) Family Support Group
67 Evendons Lane
Wokingham
Berkshire RG11 4AD
(Tel. 01734 770258)

Aims and provisions: lectures and information on syndrome; contact with families.

Retinitis pigmentosa

ALTERNATIVE NAMES

Rod-cone dystrophy; pigmentary retinal degeneration.

INCIDENCE

There is a group of conditions all classified under the name of retinitis pigmentosa. These all have a similar pathology in the retina – the light sensitive layer at the back of the eye. Modes of inheritance, severity and the age of onset of symptoms are the distinguishing factors between the different types.

Retinitis pigmentosa is also a feature of some other syndromes, such as one of the mucopolysaccharide diseases (Hunter's syndrome, for example) or Usher's syndrome, which can also have retinitis pigmentosa as part of the problems encountered in their particular syndrome. Between one person in every 2000 and every 7000 is thought to be affected. Many of these people will have only minor visual problems; these can include poor night vision.

Both boys and girls can be affected, with the exception of the X-linked form of retinitis pigmentosa, which affects only boys. Antenatal diagnosis is not routinely available at present.

CAUSATION

There appear to be three distinct modes of inheritance of retinitis pigmentosa. Autosomal recessive, autosomal dominant and an X-linked recessive form have all been described. As well as these inheritance patterns around half the cases of retinitis pigmentosa are the sole members of the family with the condition.

The autosomal recessive type appears to be the most common. This type first gives rise to symptoms during the first 20 years of life and progresses until the fifties or sixties when there is often severe visual loss.

The autosomal dominant type can appear early in the teenage years, but more frequently begins to give problems later in life, around 40 to 50 years of age. Progress is slower in this type.

The X-linked form is the least common and, of course, only affects boys. This type is frequently the most severe and there will be severe visual disability by middle age.

These different types are thought to arise from different gene defects.

CHARACTERISTICS

The basic abnormality in retinitis pigmentosa is a relative decrease in the number of 'rods' and 'cones' in the retina. These rods and cones are the light receptors which are a vital stage in the process of normal vision. In addition, clumps of pigmented tissue can be seen in the retina. The tiny blood vessels of the retina also show degenerative changes.

All these changes add up, from a clinical point of view, to **reduced vision**. The amount by which vision is reduced is very variable and some people will manage quite adequately, with only reduced night, and peripheral, vision. Often the first hint that a child may have retinitis pigmentosa is a complaint that he/she cannot see as well in the dark as his/her playfellows. A further sign is a narrowing of the amount that can be seen peripherally. (People with normal vision probably do not realize just how much they rely on their peripheral vision to make sense of the world around them. It is not until this is lost and virtual 'tunnel' vision becomes the result, that its importance is obvious.) **Colour vision** is, at times, also affected.

Retinitis pigmentosa is not associated with other abnormalities elsewhere in the body. The exception is, of course, when retinitis pigmentosa is part of other syndromes such as Usher's syndrome or one of the mucopolysaccharide syndromes.

MANAGEMENT IMPLICATIONS

Young children will not show any effects of their retinitis pigmentosa if they have the condition. But at around ten to 12 years of age their vision will deteriorate. Complaints of being unable to see the television or the blackboard at school clearly may be the first intimation that the child has a pigmented retina. Referral to an ophthalmologist will confirm the diagnosis when the retina is visualized with an ophthalmoscope.

Comprehensive vision testing is necessary to see if there is any degree of short-sight. This, and any other, refractive errors can be corrected by appropriate lenses, but no spectacles can help the basic problem in the retina.

Regular tests of vision throughout life are necessary to determine the rate of progress of the condition. In many cases this progression is slow and only in advanced years is blindness the result. A few children, however, may need special schooling facilities for their poor vision.

There are night vision aids available which can help with this aspect of retinitis pigmentosa.

In the USA, trials with vitamin supplements have been undertaken. There has been some suggestion that this treatment may slow the progression of the disease, but no conclusive proof has been demonstrated as yet.

THE FUTURE

Careers which rely heavily on excellent vision, such as airline pilots, will not be possible for people with retinitis pigmentosa. But apart from those people who suffer from the severe, and rapidly progressive form, most careers will be possible. Life expectancy is normal for the retinitis pigmentosa sufferer. It is only when the condition is associated with some other, more serious, aspect (as found in other syndromes), that life expectancy is reduced.

SELF-HELP GROUPS

British Retinitis Pigmentosa Society
Pond House
Lillingstone
Dayrell
Buckinghamshire MK18 5AS
(Tel. 01280 860363)

Aims and provisions: information booklets available; fund-raising for research.
The following group will also be able to give advice and help:

The Royal National Institute for the Blind
224 Great Portland Street
London WIN 6AA
(Tel. 0171 388 1266)

Rett's syndrome

INCIDENCE

Rett's syndrome is thought to occur in approximately one in every 10 000 to 12 000 female births, but recent research has shown that the condition is probably more common than was hitherto thought. It is now considered to be one of the commoner causes of retardation in girls. The condition seems, at present, only to affect girls, there having been no confirmed male cases.

So far, there have been no biochemical or physiological abnormalities detected during life. Diagnosis is, therefore, entirely clinical. Definitive criteria have been agreed internationally.

HISTORY

The syndrome was first described by Dr Andreas Rett from Vienna in 1966. There are a number of centres throughout the world that are now collaborating in research into this syndrome.

CAUSATION

At present, the mode of inheritance is uncertain, but as only girls are affected, it would appear that there may be mutation of a gene on the X chromosome. The present hypothesis is that this abnormality is incompatible with life in the male embryo.

From post-mortem studies, the brain appears to be surprisingly normal, with no degenerative or storage disease apparent. But there is suspicion that certain areas in the cortex and basal ganglia may be affected. Evidence suggests that Rett's syndrome is a primary genetic disorder which only comes to light as development proceeds. This hypothesis fits the clinical picture. It is thought that some defect in the metabolism of noradrenaline and dopamine may cause this syndrome.

CHARACTERISTICS

Following a normal pregnancy and birth, the baby develops within the accepted range of normal until around nine to 12 months, when **development ceases**. At this stage, the baby may be floppy, placid and show jerky movements. Then a period of regression sets in, with loss of the skills already learned. This stage may last for weeks only, but can persist for many months.

Speech: single words are usually developed, although it is rare for two or more words to be put together. During the regressive stage, these skills disappear.

Physical motor skills of both large and fine movements will be progressively lost. Walking becomes stiff and clumsy. Children previously able to feed themselves will lose this skill. As well as this loss of voluntary movement, involuntary hand movements such as frequent clapping, wringing and squeezing are very characteristic of Rett's syndrome.

Later, there is a tendency for **muscle wasting** to occur. Deformities of the spine and lower limbs can develop, with increased muscle tone. Some girls become chair-bound, but many women and girls can walk independently. Scoliosis can be made worse as a result of wasted muscles and a sedentary life style.

These facts point to some disturbance in the central organization of movement in the brain.

Breathing: in many girls the breathing pattern is disturbed with hyperventilation alternating with periods of breath-holding. During these periods of disturbed breathing the involuntary movements of the hands are seen to increase.

Epilepsy may also occur. Abnormalities are seen on the EEG tracing and are particularly in evidence in young girls when breathing is normal. This unusual finding is characteristic of Rett's syndrome.

Learning disability is profound, and stable from around five years of age. The child is left with no speech and few self-help skills. Some communication can occur. Eye contact is good and girls will respond to conversation.

Periods of crying are common during the regression stage, but usually decrease with age.

MANAGEMENT IMPLICATIONS

Epilepsy: various drugs may have to be tried to control seizures if these are troublesome. Several different drugs, or a combination of drugs may need to be given before a suitable one is found. Changes in the drug therapy may also be needed over time.

Learning disability: children with Rett's syndrome will need assessment and subsequent admittance to schools for severe learning difficulties. Reassessment must be carried out on a regular basis to ensure that new needs can be met. Positive therapy in the form of structured training in life skills must be undertaken to prevent further deterioration.

Relative immobility can sometimes lead to **contractures** in joints. Physiotherapy is useful in the prevention of this. Hydrotherapy is valuable and children enjoy this form of treatment.

All methods of **communication** should be tried. From ten years of age communication skills can be seen to improve in some children. Thus, it is important that all possible channels of communication are kept open. It must be remembered that although sight and hearing appear to be normal in the Rett's syndrome girl, reaction times are slow. So, patience, understanding and a quiet environment are necessary to enable maximum benefit from skills training.

Music therapy has been found to be successful in controlling some of the extraneous movements of the hands, such as wringing, clapping, etc. Dr Rett has worked extensively with children in this area of therapy.

THE FUTURE

Children with Rett's syndrome commonly survive into their early forties. Occasionally, some deaths occur suddenly and unexpectedly in midchildhood.

Unfortunately, an independent life is never possible for sufferers from Rett's syndrome. But with careful supervision and behavioural training, a reasonable lifestyle can be attained.

Families, too, will need constant advice and support if the child is to stay in her home environment. Rett's syndrome is particularly distressing, as early development is normal. Day centres and respite care can do much to support families.

SELF-HELP GROUPS

UK Rett Syndrome Association
Hartspool
Golden Valley
Castlemorton
Malvern
Worcestershire WR13 6AA
(Tel. 01684 833357)

Aims and provisions: to offer families and carers support and friendship; to influence professionals and to further progress in fields of education, treatment and understanding of Rett's syndrome; to assist in research projects.

National Rett Syndrome Association
15 Tanzie-Knowe Drive
Camberlang
Glasgow G72 8RG
(Tel. 0141 641 7662)

Reye's syndrome

ALTERNATIVE NAMES

Reye's fatty liver syndrome; Reye's disease.

INCIDENCE

In the early 1970s there were reports of a specific condition in infants and young children which, if they survived the original serious illness, could result in permanent disability. Subsequently, much more has been learnt about the natural history of the disease. The number of children suffering from disability due to this cause is not accurately known. In recent years, the incidence is thought to be decreasing. Children of any age, from infancy to around 19 years can be affected. The younger age group have been seen to be more at risk. All races and both sexes can be affected by Reye's syndrome.

HISTORY

Reye's syndrome was first described by an Australian pathologist, Dr Douglas Reye.

CAUSATION

Reye's syndrome follows on from an acute viral infection, such as an upper respiratory tract infection, chickenpox, flu or a diarrhoreal illness. Various viruses have been implicated in these forerunning infections.

The use of aspirin to control fever and pain in young children with an infection has been suggested to be an added causative factor in Reye's syndrome. About 60% of children with Reye's syndrome have taken aspirin before the onset of the acute illness. As a result of this, aspirin is no longer prescribed for the relief of pain and fever in children under 12 years of age.

Recent research has suggested that some children who develop Reye's syndrome have an underlying genetically determined metabolic defect. This predisposes them to the symptoms seen in Reye's syndrome following an acute infection.

CHARACTERISTICS

The **acute illness** is one in which persistent vomiting and convulsions follow on from an often mild everyday infection. The child becomes irritable and may be aggressive. He/she is confused and lacking in energy. Eventually, drowsiness can lead on to delirium and coma with a potentially fatal outcome. Bleeding from the stomach can also follow on from the persistent vomiting. Abnormal fatty deposits are to be found in the liver in association with encephalopathy (changes in the brain as a result of the illness) at post-mortem. The diagnosis can be difficult, as Reye's syndrome can closely mimic encephalitis, meningitis or acute poisoning, for example. The child with any of these serious infections will, of course, need hospital treatment. Liver function and blood-clotting tests are necessary to confirm the clinical diagnosis.

The chronic phase: if the child survives the acute illness, recovery can be complete with no remaining permanent disability. Unfortunately, some children will be left with a varying degree of brain damage. This may be only slight, but regrettably severe learning disability can occur. If the infection affects babies under one year of age, there is more likelihood of residual disability than if this syndrome affects children over this age.

MANAGEMENT IMPLICATIONS

Acute phase: urgent emergency treatment is necessary to reduce the risk of permanent brain damage. Early intensive treatment has been shown to increase the chance of survival and also to decrease the risk of permanent brain damage. Intensive care facilities in hospital are frequently necessary in this acute phase.

Chronic phase: the acute stage of Reye's syndrome is a serious illness. The young sufferer will need several weeks of convalescence before he/she is fully fit again. Adequate rest, with a nourishing diet and graded physical activity will be needed. Many children will recover completely from their acute infection and suffer no long-term after effects, but regrettably some children will be left with permanent residual damage. The degree will vary, but in some cases learning disability will be severe. If there is any doubt at all regarding possible brain damage resulting from the original illness, multidisciplinary assessment will be needed. From the results of such assessment, any specific disability is unearthed, and help can be given where necessary. In the most severely affected children, special educational facilities will be needed. Careful developmental follow-up over the succeeding years will be necessary. Any problem with movement, speech or cognitive function will need specialized help from the appropriate therapists. It is difficult to be more specific, as the after-effects of this illness are so variable.

THE FUTURE

This will depend very much on the severity of the disability left once the acute illness is over. Recovery can be complete, with no sequelae. Alternatively, varying degrees of disability can remain, affecting the remainder of the child's life. If this is the case, sheltered accommodation and work after special schooling facilities will be necessary.

SELF-HELP GROUP

National Reye's Syndrome Foundation of the UK
15 Nicholas Gardens
Pyrford
Woking
Surrey GU2 8SD
(Tel. 01932 346843)

Aims and provisions: support for parents; inform public and medical profession; raise funds for research to find the cause, develop early detection and improve treatment methods.

Riley–Day syndrome

ALTERNATIVE NAME

Dysautonomia.

INCIDENCE

This is rare in general populations. The Riley–Day syndrome is largely confined to Ashkenazi Jewish families. The incidence in these families is relatively high, being found in approximately one in every 3700 births. About one person in every 100 carries the gene. Boys and girls can be affected equally.

The Riley–Day syndrome primarily affects the autonomic nervous system, which controls the involuntary actions of the body and functions such as blood pressure and temperature. In addition, some voluntary movements, such as speech, swallowing and other physical movements can also be affected.

CAUSATION

Riley–Day syndrome is inherited as an autosomal recessive. The incidence is relatively high in the population at special risk due to the comparatively closed community, with intermarriage being common. There is no ante-natal diagnosis possible at present. Genetic counselling is advisable for families who already have a member with the condition.

CHARACTERISTICS

It is only the clumping together of a number of fairly non-specific symptoms in a child with a family history of the disorder that can lead to suspicions of the Riley–Day syndrome being present. All children with the syndrome have the following features:

No **tears** are ever shed by a child with the Riley–Day syndrome. This absence of tears can lead to ulceration of the cornea. Although there is some minimal tear formation in the tear glands, this is so defective as to leave no tears available to overflow onto the cheeks during everyday upsets.

The **tongue** in the child with the Riley–Day syndrome is smooth due to the absence of the papillae which are normally seen.

Other common signs affect up to 95% of children with the Riley–Day syndrome.

Blotching of the skin, due to the primary disorder in the autonomic system which controls the contraction and dilatation of the blood vessels. This is particularly noticeable when the child is excited.

Temperature control, also regulated by the autonomic nervous system, is unstable, and can become dangerously high or low. Excessive sweating, in an endeavour to lower a high temperature, is frequently seen in these children.

Pain is not felt as acutely as normal. This might seem like an advantage, but pain has the function of giving warning of injury or disease so that action can be taken to avoid further damage. If this in-built warning system does not function adequately, injuries can continue and disease processes can become dangerously advanced before treatment is given. The ability to distinguish between heat and cold is also often diminished – again increasing the risk of injury.

Inco-ordination of limbs when performing everyday activities is also noticeable in the child with the Riley–Day syndrome. In addition, an unsteady gait is often seen.

Speech can also be adversely affected by the relative inco-ordination of the muscles of tongue and throat.

Scoliosis, together with general poor growth can also be a problem.

Intelligence is usually normal in children with the Riley–Day syndrome, but emotional instability is common, with wild swings of mood from elation to misery.

Blood pressure control can also be unreliable. Hypotension is especially likely to occur when the child gets up from a lying or sitting position. This can cause temporary loss of consciousness at times.

Other less common, but nevertheless important, features include **swallowing difficulties** in infancy. This can make feeding a problem in the early days of life. **Uncontrollable vomiting** can also add to the problems of adequate nutrition in this age group of Riley-Day sufferers. Inhalation pneumonia is an ever-present threat when these two problems are encountered in infancy.

MANAGEMENT IMPLICATIONS

Eyes: extra special care must be taken to protect the eyes of children with the Riley–Day syndrome. Dust which would normally be washed away by tears can cause serious abrasions on the cornea, with possible subsequent ulceration. Therefore, any foreign body in the eye must be treated with extreme care. Treatment with adequate washing out of the foreign body together with greasy, antibiotic ointment is a necessary precaution.

Infections of any kind must also receive adequate and early treatment, due to the instability of temperature control. This lack of control predisposes the child to febrile convulsions, so cooling measures must be taken as well as treatment of the underlying cause of the fever.

Pain insensitivity must be mentioned to teachers when schooldays are reached so that watch can be kept for any potentially damaging incidents.

Speech therapy is valuable in helping the inco-ordinated muscle function of lips, tongue and throat.

Behaviour modification techniques may be of value in controlling the **emotional instability** which can be so destructive a part of the behaviour pattern of these children. The help of a clinical psychologist can do much to improve life for the child and his/her family. During anaesthesia, care must be taken with drugs which exert an effect on the autonomic nervous system.

THE FUTURE

Children with the Riley–Day syndrome often succumb in early childhood to the effects of the swallowing difficulties which are part of their pathology – inhalation pneumonia often being the result. This can also recur in early adult life, with similar fatal results. Career prospects will be limited due to infections, possible poor vision due to previous unrecognized corneal abrasions and also to the emotional liability so frequently seen in people with this syndrome.

SELF-HELP GROUP

Dysautonomia Society of Great Britain
2 Oakwood Avenue
Borehamwood
Hertfordshire WO6 1SR
(Tel. 0181 953 5900)

Aims and provisions: help with nursing problems; fund-raising for research.

Rubinstein–Taybi syndrome

INCIDENCE

This is a rare disorder, the incidence of which was reported to be only three affected in 100 000. This report related to the province of Ontario in Canada. Nevertheless, it has been estimated that as many as one in every 500 people in institutions for those with severe learning disability are affected by the Rubinstein–Taybi syndrome. This makes this syndrome a not insignificant cause of severe learning disability. Because of the variability of the characteristics seen in this syndrome, the diagnosis can, at times, be made only tentatively. This further adds to the difficulties in assessing the incidence of the Rubinstein–Taybi syndrome.

The condition has been reported from many countries, including Japan and Africa as well as populations of Caucasian origin. Both sexes can be equally affected.

CAUSATION

The inheritance pattern of the Rubinstein–Taybi syndrome is uncertain at present. It may have an environmental cause as well as a genetic predisposition, or there may be a genetic cause as yet undetermined. Several sets of twins with the condition have been reported and other familial connections are known. These facts would make some genetic inheritance more likely.

There is no antenatal test available to detect the condition.

CHARACTERISTICS

Developmental delay is apparent in all children with the Rubinstein–Taybi syndrome. The delay affects all aspects of development, both mental and physical. The degree of delay varies from child to child, but the IQ will not be above 60 in the child with this condition. Along with the learning disability goes varying degrees of language delay.

Microcephaly (head circumference at, or below, the lower range of normal). The head circumference measurement is an excellent indicator of brain growth, so it follows that all children with a head circumference smaller than usual will have some degree of learning disability.

Physical growth in children with this syndrome is also retarded. Final height at 18 years of age will only be on the 50th centile of the standard growth charts.

There are a number of unusual **facial features** associated with the Rubinstein–Taybi syndrome, which make the children comparatively easy to recognize. **Eyes** are widely set apart, and eyelids have a characteristic drooping appearance (ptosis). **Eyelashes** are often beautifully long. **Squints** are also common, as are **refractive errors**. The child's **nose** is an especially obvious feature, being on the large side and convex in a typical Romanesque manner. The mouth is small with, typically, a **high, arched palate**. **Teeth** are also often overcrowded, with an incomplete 'bite'.

Finger and **toe** features are among the most frequently found characteristics. Both thumbs, and nearly always both great toes, are broad and flattened at the ends. The great toes are also widely separated from the other toes of the foot (cf Down's syndrome). Occasionally, the terminal bones of thumbs and big toes are bifid, this feature adding to the broad, spatulate aspect of these digits. Other fingers can also be broader than usual at the ends. Toes can also overlap each other.

Other **skeletal problems** can also occur. For example, unusual construction of the lower vertebrae gives rise to an awkward gait.

In boys with this syndrome, undescended **testes** are frequently found.

Many children also have excess **hair** on their bodies.

There are a number of other abnormalities that can be associated with the Rubinstein–Taybi syndrome, including **heart defects**, **renal problems**, **convulsions** and **flame-shaped naevi** on foreheads or backs of necks. It is unusual for all these features to be found in one individual, but they occur with sufficient regularity to make remembrance of them necessary when caring for a child with this syndrome.

MANAGEMENT IMPLICATIONS

Developmental delay, and all its educational and social effects, must be assessed and regularly monitored by a multidisciplinary team. Particular areas of delay, such as speech, should receive appropriate therapy. Early teaching of self-help skills will help to give a better quality of life to both the affected child and his/her family.

Appropriate **schooling**, geared to the child's assessed abilities, will be necessary when school age is reached. Depending on local facilities, either a special school or a unit with appropriately resourced facilities will nearly always be necessary for the child with the Rubinstein–Taybi syndrome.

Squints and **refractive errors** (be they short-sight or long-sight with or without astigmatism) must be assessed and treated appropriately. Squints may need surgery to prevent amblyopia. Refractive errors, more common in children with this syndrome than in the general childhood population, will need corrective lenses. Most children with these errors, whatever their learning disability, will willingly wear their spectacles. They appreciate the added dimension of clear vision.

Undescended **testes** will need operative procedures to bring these organs down into the correct position in the scrotum. Malignant change or damage due to trauma are both risks if this is not done.

Surgery may also be necessary on **toes** if the big toe is so large and displaced as to give rise to difficulties in finding suitable shoes.

Children with the Rubinstein–Taybi syndrome can suffer from **urinary tract infections** more frequently than their peers. This is particularly the case if there are associated renal abnormalities. These infections must be recognized and treated with the appropriate antibiotic when they occur.

Convulsions, if they occur, must also be treated with anti-convulsant drugs.

Obesity can be an added problem in the later childhood years. This should receive dietetic advice and monitoring.

Teeth, if overcrowding and/or malocclusion are present, should receive dental care.

THE FUTURE

Most children with the Rubinstein–Taybi syndrome will never be able to lead a fully independent life due to their learning disability. Full-time care will be necessary for practically all individuals. Lifespan is thought to be within the normal range as long as there are no potentially life-threatening heart or renal abnormalities present.

A specific type of brain tumour is more common in people with this syndrome and this can have fatal consequences.

SELF-HELP GROUPS

Rubinstein–Taybi Syndrome Support Group
46 Windsor Road
Great Harwood
Blackburn
Lancashire BB6 7RR
(Tel. 01254 889122)

Aims and provisions: contact with other families; information on the condition; newsletter.

San Filippo syndrome

ALTERNATIVE NAME

Mucopolysaccharidosis 3.

INCIDENCE

San Filippo syndrome is one of the mucopolysaccharide diseases. The mucopolysaccharides are complex sugars. The defect in San Filippo syndrome is a lack, or deficiency of, a specific enzyme which breaks down one of these complex sugars. Due to this, there is an accumulation of the particular sugar in the organs and tissues. It is this build-up which causes the signs and symptoms of the disease. There are at least four sub-types of this syndrome, but all are similar clinically. The sub-types are known as San Filippo A, B, C and D. The difference between these four types is in the actual enzyme involved. San Filippo A is the most common.

Around one in 25 000 live births exhibit this enzyme deficiency. Boys and girls are equally affected.

HISTORY

With advanced biochemical techniques, the specific enzyme defects which occur in all the mucopolysaccharidoses have been found. All these diseases have a similar clinical picture, with greater emphasis on certain specific signs and symptoms in each syndrome, due to the specific sugar metabolism affected. (See Hunter's, Hurler's and Morquio's syndromes.)

CAUSATION

San Filippo syndrome is inherited as an autosomal recessive genetic defect. Even though the enzyme for each sub-type is different the end result is that excess heparin sulphate is excreted and also stored in large amounts in the body due to the deficiency of the specific enzyme.

The condition can be identified antenatally by chorionic villus sampling at around the tenth week of pregnancy.

CHARACTERISTICS

Children with San Filippo syndrome are normal at birth and initial developmental milestones are within the normal range. At around two to three years of age, or maybe even later – at early school age, this normal developmental progress slows.

Mental and motor development: sadly, after the initial normal growth and development in all areas, between the ages of two and five years, there is rapid decline both mentally and physically. Most self-help skills and intellectual ability are quickly lost. The child becomes agitated and upset by the smallest changes in routine. Bizarre behaviour patterns are also noticed, similar to those seen in older severely demented people. Within a relatively short time he/she is confined to bed due to his/her inability to walk or to control his/her movements adequately.

Sleep disturbances can often be a distressing feature of the San Filippo syndrome. Parents can become quite exhausted by their baby's unusual sleep pattern, which includes frequent waking during the night.

Growth is slowed at the same time as the mental and motor skills are lost. Although the gross short stature of Hunter's and Hurler's syndromes is not seen, children with San Filippo syndrome rarely grow beyond the 25th centile on the standard growth charts.

Facial features: there is a mild coarsening of the features in a similar way to that seen in the other mucopolysccharide diseases, although this is not as marked as in the other diseases with a similar background. The tongue and lips become enlarged out of proportion with the rest of the face, and head size also increases.

Frequent **upper respiratory tract infections** are also a feature of babies with this syndrome. This can, of course, add to the sleeping problems as the baby is distressed by his/her blocked nose and all the other unpleasant symptoms of a head cold.

Deafness is thought to occur later in childhood, due most probably to the frequent upper respiratory tract infections. Hearing can be difficult to check accurately due to the severe learning disabilites from which San Filippo children suffer.

Joints: as in the other mucopolysaccharide diseases there is some restriction in the movements of the joints. This, together with the loss of other motor skills, leads to lack of mobility.

All these signs and symptoms can be directly traced to the accumulation of the specific complex sugar which is continually being laid down in the tissue, and particularly in the central nervous system in San Filippo syndrome.

MANAGEMENT IMPLICATIONS

Once the diagnosis has been made with certainty, parents should be sensitively counselled as to the future. It is incredibly hard to watch your seemingly normal baby deteriorate in all ways so rapidly and completely. Parents will need to be helped through the normal bereavement processes – denial, anger, guilt and final acceptance, for the loss of a normal child is as truly a bereavement as if the child had died.

Learning disability: the first sign of the occurrence of the regression from continuing normal development is often unusual and unpredictably inappropriate behaviour. The formerly biddable child will not be amenable to following the normal well-established routine of the household and will exhibit temper tantrums for no obvious reason. Previously well-known and practised self-help skills, such as feeding and toileting, will be lost.

During this stage, patience and understanding are vital, and parents will need to be helped through each problem as it arises. Respite care for short or longer periods of time are essential in order that parents can have a break to recharge their own batteries as well as to give a little time to the rest of their family. Eventually, schooling for severely disabled children will be necessary.

Attempts to assess **hearing** should be made. This in itself can prove difficult, and even if it is thought that hearing aids would prove to be beneficial, it is unlikely that the child will tolerate them.

THE FUTURE

The outlook for children with San Filippo syndrome is bleak. Death usually occurs before the age of 20 is reached, the sufferer being bed-ridden in a severely demented state.

There have been attempts to replace the missing enzyme, but so far this has proved to be unsuccessful.

SELF-HELP GROUP

Society for Mucopolysaccharide Diseases
55 Hill Avenue
Amersham
Buckinghamshire HP6 5BX
(Tel. 01494 434156)

Aims and provisions: support and advice for parents; raises funds for research, including grants; annual parent weekend conference; supplies specialized hospital equipment; booklets and leaflets produced.

Sickle cell anaemia

INCIDENCE

Sickle cell anaemia (as with thalassaemia, which is also an inherited blood condition) is only seen in certain racial groups. These include populations around the Mediterranean – areas of Greece, southern Turkey and Italy. Definitive areas of West Africa and southern India also show a high incidence of this inherited disorder, as do a high percentage (up to 40%) of black Americans. In this latter group it is thought that the incidence can be as high as one in every 625 births. Both sexes are equally affected.

If the parents are known to be carriers of this condition, antenatal tests can be done on the unborn baby.

In various parts of Britain with a high immigrant population, the incidence of sickle cell anaemia is high. Special clinics to deal especially with this condition have been set up in many places.

HISTORY

It has been found that certain people with sickle cell anaemia have some protection against the ravages of a particularly virulent form of malaria – a common condition in parts of the world where sickle cell anaemia is also found. (It is a debatable point as to which condition is preferable!)

CAUSATION

Sickle cell anaemia is inherited as an autosomal recessive condition.

There is a 'carrier' state for sickle cell disease. This is known as the 'sickle cell trait'. Whilst people with this trait do not have any signs and symptoms of the disease, it is important that their medical practitioners are aware of their genetic inheritance. Special care will be needed during anaesthetics and certain surgical procedures, but apart from this, these people should be firmly reassured that their sickle cell trait will have no effect at all on their daily lives.

The basic problem in this condition is an abnormality on the structure of haemoglobin (the oxygen-carrying substance in the red blood cells). Haemoglobin is an extremely complex substance. In view of this, a number of problems can arise, and 'sickling' of the red blood cells is just one of these. Thalassaemia is a further condition affecting haemoglobin. Due to the abnormality in the haemoglobin in sickle cell anaemia, the red blood cells themselves are distorted from their normal smooth elliptical shape to an elongate 'sickle' shaped one. It is this unusual shape that is responsible for some of the symptoms of the disease. The particular type of anaemia accounts for the manifestations of the disease.

It is important that the diagnosis of the exact type of haemaglobinopathy (diseases of abnormal blood production) is made as soon as possible, so that the appropriate treatment and care can be given.

CHARACTERISTICS

The first indications that sickle cell anaemia is present can occur when the affected baby is around six months of age. At this time, swellings on the short **bones** of hands and/or feet will be noticed. The baby can also be feverish and irritable. These typical swellings are a direct result of the 'clumping' of the abnormal red blood cells in the small blood vessels of this area of the body. The growing bone is damaged and responds by an overgrowth of new bone. Infection may, or may not, play a part in this early manifestation of sickle cell anaemia.

In older children and adults, painful **crises**, usually accompanied by a fever, occur when the distorted red blood cells clump together. Any part of the body can be affected – kidneys, liver, lungs or brain, for example.

As a result of this clumping together of the red blood cells, the blood supply is reduced – or cut off altogether – to the affected organ of the body. The symptoms suffered will be related to whichever organ or tissue is involved. For example, renal failure may develop if the blood vessels of the kidney are severely affected. Similarly, paralysis of one side of the body can occur if the blood vessels in the brain are blocked by clumps of abnormally shaped red blood cells.

These crises are frequently precipitated by bouts of infection. It is, therefore, vitally important that infections in children with sickle cell anaemia are treated with a degree of urgency.

Strenuous exercise can also lead to a crisis occurring, due to the extra need for oxygen not being met by the abnormal red blood cells containing insufficient amounts of this vital gas.

Anaesthetics will also need to be given with care to sufferers from sickle cell anaemia.

Anaemia, in which the child will be listless, pale and maybe breathless on any exertion, is a persistent hazard for sufferers from this condition. Exacerbations in the anaemic state occur in episodes which are thought to be related to a specific type of viral infection. Again, the anaemia is a direct result of the lack of oxygen carrying power of the abnormal haemo-globin on the red blood cells.

The **spleen**, tucked away up under the left lower ribs and intimately concerned with red blood cell production and destruction, can also give rise to specific problems. There can be a sudden onset of severe anaemia with a greatly enlarged painful spleen. This is known as a 'sequestration' crisis, and mainly affects babies and younger children. The sufferer will collapse and need urgent hospital treatment. Transfusion of blood under these circumstances may be necessary to save life.

Children with sickle cell anaemia do seem to be especially prone to **osteomyelitis** (an infection in the bones of any part of the body). The reason for this is unclear, but any pain localized to a particular bone must be fully investigated.

Enuresis (day-time or night-time wetting) can also be a problem. This can persist into adult life and is due to the kidneys being unable to concentrate the urine properly, so that large quantities of dilute urine need to be passed from the bladder at frequent intervals.

INVESTIGATIONS

Specialized blood tests on both child and parents will confirm the diagnosis of sickle cell anaemia. It is important that sickle cell anaemia is differen-tiated from other somewhat similar conditions, as both treatment and outcome are different.

MANAGEMENT IMPLICATIONS

One of the most important aspects of the care of the child with sickle cell anaemia is to **educate** and **alert** the parents in the recognition of the crises that can occur. It can be all too easy to think that abdominal or chest pain is due to some relatively trivial childhood condition, when in reality the child is suffering from a flare-up of the inherited condition. Obviously, if other members of the immediate family also suffer from sickle cell anae-mia, parents will be more easily able to recognize the symptoms attribu-table to the disease.

Parents should also be taught to recognize the dangerous crises affecting the spleen. This will show itself as acute abdominal pain with the tender spleen being easy to feel in the left upper part of the abdomen. Under these circumstances the need for urgent medical attention should be impressed on the parents.

Each bout of **infection**, of whatever type, must be treated quickly and adequately in an attempt to avoid a crisis due to the sickle cell anaemia. In young children prophylactic treatment with penicillin by mouth has proved effective in preventing serious infections such as those caused by the pneumococcus bacteria.

If a **crisis** does occur, pain relieving drugs are necessary, together with plenty to drink. Many of these events can be successfully managed at home if parents fully understand how important it is that their child should have copious fluids and adequate pain relieving drugs. Severe attacks will need hospital admission for intravenous fluids to be given. Specific antibiotics will also be necessary to counteract the infection.

Blood transfusion can also be necessary at times to counteract the severe anaemia which can occur.

A particular type of infection with a parvo-virus – giving rise to a 'flu-like illness – can have deleterious effects on the bone-marrow. Red cell production is reduced by this infection and can result in severe anaemia.

An adequate nutritionally sound **diet** during childhood can help to reduce to a minimum the above serious manifestations of the disease. It is also important that children with sickle cell anaemia should not become exhausted and/or over-heated by strenuous physical exercise.

Schooling in mainstream schools is possible as long as teaching staff understand the need for immediate assessment and treatment if the child should complain of severe pain in any part of the body. The dangers of physical over-exertion should also be stressed under these conditions.

Absences – sometimes frequent – from school can undermine the education of the child with sickle cell anaemia. Good liaison between home and school, with possible work sent home to do when the child feels well enough, can do much to minimize problems of this nature.

Bone-marrow transplantation has been carried out in a few children and has proved to be successful and curative.

Certain **drugs** have also recently been researched in an effort to reduce adverse symptoms, with some success.

THE FUTURE

It is difficult to predict the outcome of sickle cell anaemia in any one individual child. Access to quick medical care is of enormous advantage and can allow the sufferer to lead a full and productive life.

Genetic counselling is advisable before a pregnancy is embarked upon.

SELF-HELP GROUPS

The Sickle Cell Society
54 Station Road
London NW10 4UA
(Tel. 0181 961 7795 and 0181 961 4006)

Aims and provisions: contact with other families; information about the condition; holiday schemes for affected children; videos; information packs; newsletter.

OSCAR (Organization for Sickle Cell Research)
Tiverton Sickle Cell Community Centre
Tiverton Road,
Tottenham
London N15 6RT
(Tel. 0181 802 3055 and 0181 802 0994)

Aims and provisions: advice on housing, welfare and social aspects of sickle cell anaemia; financial assistance; educational talks to community groups; booklets and leaflets on specific aspects of the disease.

Silver–Russell syndrome

ALTERNATIVE NAMES

Silver syndrome; dwarfism – Silver–Russell type.

INCIDENCE

The exact incidence of this syndrome is not known, but cases have been reported from many parts of the world. All races and ethnic groups seem to be susceptible and both boys and girls seem to be affected equally. (However, there has been an X-linked Silver syndrome described, which has similar characteristics, but which, due to the mode of inheritance, affects boys only.)

HISTORY

This syndrome was described by both Dr Silver and Dr Russell in the 1950s. Further work regarding specific aspects of the syndrome was reported in 1964.

CAUSATION

At present, the mode of inheritance is not clear. Either an autosomal recessive inheritance or a dominant inheritance with incomplete penetrance has been postulated. Suggestions have been made that placental insufficiency may be a factor in the aetiology of this syndrome. This lack of adequate functioning of the placenta may in itself be an inherited characteristic.

CHARACTERISTICS

Short stature: babies with the Silver–Russell syndrome are born smaller than normal. Growth throughout childhood usually follows along the normal growth lines but at, or below, the third centile on the growth charts. A few children have been reported to show a 'catch-up' growth spurt around puberty so that their final adult height more nearly approaches the norm, but this is unusual.

Asymmetry is seen, involving either one complete half of the child's body, or a particular part – a limb or part of the skull, for example. The degree of asymmetry varies markedly from child to child. Often, this aspect of the condition is not noticed at birth or during the early months of life. It is only later, when growth proceeds at a rapid rate, that the unusual development is noticed.

Advanced sexual development, particularly in girls, is a common feature of the Silver–Russell syndrome. Breast development, menstruation and adult distribution of hair can all occur earlier than is usual. These effects go alongside elevated levels of gonadotrophins in the blood and urine.

The shape of the **head** is also a noticeable characteristic among children with the Silver–Russell syndrome. Foreheads are wide and taper down to a thin pointed chin, giving the appearance of a triangular shaped face. One further feature of interest is that the anterior fontanelle tends to be later than usual in closing.

The **hands** of children with the Silver–Russell syndrome are characteristic in as much as they frequently have an inturning little finger (cf Down's syndrome). Toes can also show minor abnormalities, such as webbing, between the second and third toes in particular.

Cafe-au-lait spots, similar to those seen in neurofibromatosis, are often seen on any part of the body. These can vary in size from those only the size of a small freckle to pigmented areas of over 30 cm in diameter.

Children with this syndrome have often been noticed to sweat excessively.

The last three characteristics (in head, fingers and skin) are all variable manifestations of the Silver–Russell syndrome. It is the combination of the short stature, asymmetry of parts of the body, the small size at birth, and the precocious sexual development that are the constant findings. The other added variable factors are, however, helpful in making a diagnosis.

MANAGEMENT IMPLICATIONS

There are two aspects of the Silver–Russell syndrome which can call for special help in childhood. The **short stature** and possible **asymmetry**of the skeleton can cause difficulties during school days. The short stature is not usually so marked that the child will need special equipment, as do children with achondroplasia. The asymmetry of the body, if severe and affecting a major proportion of the body, may need to be corrected with special shoes, for example, to aid normal movement. Physiotherapy is valuable in helping the youngster use the appropriate muscles correctly to balance his/her asymmetry.

The **precocious puberty** may be upsetting to both child and parents. Sensitive explanation, and practical help in school to deal with the every-day aspects of menstruation, will help the child come to terms with her unusual sexual development. It is not much fun being different from your peers in the upper junior school.

THE FUTURE

The degree of affected movement will depend very much upon the position and severity of the skeletal asymmetry and career choices may be limited by this aspect of the Silver–Russell syndrome. People with this syndrome can expect a normal lifespan.

SELF-HELP GROUPS

Silver–Russell Support Group
'Squirrels'
17 King Street Lane
Winnersh
Wokingham
Berkshire RG11 5AP
(Tel. 01734 773272 (evenings))

Aims and provisions: support via telephone and meetings.

The Child Growth Foundation
2 Mayfield Avenue
London W4 lPW
(Tel. 0181 994 7625)

This group is also able to give advice and information.

Sjorgen–Larsson syndrome

INCIDENCE

Although this is a very rare syndrome, it has been reported as occurring in many countries. Extensive research into this syndrome was done in Sweden in the 1950s. In a particular region of this country the incidence of the condition, named after the two Swedes who performed the research, was found to be around eight people in 100 000. Both boys and girls can be affected.

There are a number of other syndromes which cause a similar skin rash, but Sjorgen–Larsson syndrome can be diagnosed quite specifically by the associated features.

CAUSATION

This syndrome is inherited as an autosomal recessive characteristic. The abnormal gene responsible has not been located as yet. Carriers of the condition can be detected by the deficiency of a substance necessary for complete oxidation of a further chemical necessary for correct metabolism.

There is no antenatal test available.

CHARACTERISTICS

Skin: the most obvious feature of Sjorgen–Larsson syndrome is the specific skin abnormality. Soon after birth the baby's skin becomes reddened. Within a few weeks this redness becomes altered to a typical fish-scale like rash (icthyosis). The skin is dry and 'scaly' to the touch. Parts of the body most severely affected are the places which approximate most closely together, for example, armpits, elbow creases, around the neck and also the lower part of the abdomen. These typical skin lesions will persist throughout life.

A further characteristic of Sjorgen–Larsson syndrome is **spasticity**. This is usually confined to the lower part of the body. As a result of this around three-quarters of the sufferers from this syndrome are confined to a wheelchair for most of their lives. Legs are stiff with increased tone in the muscles. An increase in muscle tone is also often seen around the mouth region. This can cause difficulties in feeding, particularly in the early days of life, and also problems with the subsequent development of speech.

Mental abilities: almost all sufferers from this syndrome have some degree of learning disability. Some children are only mildly disabled, having an IQ level of between 70 and 90. (This level is defined as 'border-line retardation'). Other children have severe learning disabilities.

These three features are those which must be demonstrated before a diagnosis of Sjorgen–Larsson syndrome is made. As mentioned before, a number of other syndromes have icthyosis as part of their pathology, but only Sjorgen–Larsson sufferers have the added characteristics of learning disability and neurological signs.

Eyes: in around half of the children with Sjorgen–Larsson syndrome there will be a degeneration of parts of the retina. This can occur as early as two years of age. If this does occur, vision will be affected to a greater or lesser degree depending on the severity and location of the retinal degeneration.

MANAGEMENT IMPLICATIONS

Skin: the dry scales of certain areas of the skin seen in this syndrome can be very uncomfortable to live with, due to the associated dryness. Soap, which has a drying quality, should be avoided when bathing children with this condition. Lactic or glycolic acid can be used to remove the dry scales gently. This will need to be done on a regular, continuing basis. Other greasy emollient creams can also be tried in an effort to reduce the dryness. The help of a dermatologist is valuable. Clothing will need to be carefully chosen so that the dry, scaly skin does not catch on fluffy fabrics. Natural fibres, such as cotton, are probably the most suitable. As they grow older, children can become acutely embarrassed by their scaly skins so unlike the beautifully smooth skins of their contemporaries. Clothing with long sleeves and high necks will do much to reduce everyday embarrassment. Teachers will need to be informed of the child's skin condition when school days are reached, so that explanations can be given to other class members when playtime arrives in the summer.

Spasticity: little can be done to relieve this tragic neurological abnormality. In the early days of life, feeding may need extra care due to the tight mouth and throat muscles. Speech, for the same reason, may show articulation difficulties. Speech therapy input from an early age will ensure that speech develops as normally as possible. If the learning disability is severe this will, of course, give rise to greater problems in this – and other – areas of development. Regrettably, children with Sjorgen–Larsson syndrome will eventually become wheelchair bound due to their neurological abnormalities. Good nursing care will be vital to prevent pressure sores.

Learning disability: it is of vital importance that routine developmental checks are done for these babies and children on a regular basis. Just because Sjorgen–Larsson syndrome has been diagnosed, this does not necessarily mean that the child will have severe learning disability; IQ may be bordering on normal. So when school days are reached it is important that the correct school for the child's abilities is chosen if he/she is to reach his/her genetic potential.

Vision: careful checks on visual acuity should be continuous throughout life. Ophthalmic examination will show if there is any retinal degeneration present. Little can be done to improve impairment to vision from this cause, but with routine checks other refractive problems of long- or short-sight or astigmatism can be corrected by appropriate lenses, reducing the visual disability to a minimum.

THE FUTURE

This is very dependent upon the severity of the neurological and learning disabilities. Life expectancy can be reduced if either of these two aspects is severe.

SELF-HELP GROUP

There is no specific self-help group in this country at present, but the following group may be a useful contact:

MENCAP
123 Golden Lane
London EC1Y 0RT
(Tel. 0171 454 0454)

Smith–Lemli–Opitz syndrome

ALTERNATIVE NAME

RHS syndrome

INCIDENCE

The incidence of this rare syndrome is estimated to be about one in 40 000. It is thought that boys and girls are equally affected. The uncertainty of both the incidence and the ratio of affected males and females is due, in part, to the greater ease with which boys with this syndrome can be identified; the genital abnormalities being seen more readily in boys.

The only antenatal test possible at present is by ultra-sound. The genital abnormalities can be detected by this method.

Genetic counselling is advisable before a further pregnancy is embarked upon.

HISTORY

The alternative name of RHS syndrome was coined from the surnames of three families with whom Dr Opitz worked.

CAUSATION

This syndrome is inherited in an autosomal recessive manner.

CHARACTERISTICS

Growth failure: This feature can be noted antenatally as well as after birth. Due to the poor growth, both in weight and height, the baby with this syndrome has a low birth weight.

The continuing failure to thrive adequately after birth is enhanced by **feeding** difficulties. The baby's muscles are weak and hypotonic, so that sucking is poor with milk frequently being regurgitated.

Facial features include a high, narrow forehead with a small head (microcephaly), a short, tip-tilted nose, frequently a cleft palate and an under-developed lower jaw. This last feature adds to the initial feeding difficulties.

Boys are seen to have **genital abnormalities**, which include a hypospadias, a small, under-developed scrotum or ambiguous genitalia in which it is difficult, at first sight, to determine the sex of the baby.

Hands and **feet** also show abnormalities. Extra fingers are seen in around 30% of babies with the Smith–Lemli–Opitz syndrome and webbing of the toes is seen in about 10%.

To a lesser extent, **heart** and **renal** defects are seen in the most severely affected babies.

Learning disability is almost always present and can vary from a moderate to a severe degree.

MANAGEMENT IMPLICATIONS

Skilled **nursing care** is vital in the early days of life in order to overcome the feeding difficulties caused by both the unusual facial features and the general hypotonia of the baby. Weight gain improves once the early months are over and the baby's muscle tone and facial features mature.

The **genital abnormalities** will need assessment and treatment by a surgeon specializing in this field. Surgery will also need to be done at a later date on boys with a hypospadias.

Similarly, extra **fingers** may also need surgery at a later date. The webbed toes do not usually cause problems, but again may need surgery later.

Any **heart** and/or **renal** problems that come to light over the first few weeks of life will need assessment and appropriate treatment.

Developmental checks will determine the level of the child's abilities over the first few years. Parents will need sensitive counselling regarding the difficulties that their son or daughter will experience as they mature.

Suitable **schooling** will need to be investigated and provided. Close liaison between health and education authorities is vital to ensure that the most suitable environment is found for the child with Smith–Lemli–Opitz syndrome.

THE FUTURE

Regretfully, around one-quarter of all affected children will die during the first two years of life, usually as a result of the heart or renal problems associated with this syndrome. An independent life is not possible for people with this syndrome.

SELF-HELP GROUP

Smith–Lemli–Opitz Contact Group
372 Warwick Road
Solihull
Warwickshire B91 1BE
(Tel. 0121 705 0188)

Aims and provisions: contact with other parents; information on the condition; newsletter.

Smith–Magenis syndrome

ALTERNATIVE NAME

Interstitial deletion of chromosome 17.

INCIDENCE

This syndrome is rare, the exact incidence being unknown. It is thought, however, that the true incidence is higher than is classified at present. More people with the condition are being identified as chromosomal analysis becomes more widespread.

The Smith–Magenis syndrome has been reported in all parts of the world. There would seem to be a higher incidence of the condition in boys than girls, although this has not been definitely reported.

CAUSATION

In all cases of this syndrome when chromosome analysis has been done, the cause has been found to be a deletion in a particular part of chromosome 17. This is thought to arise sporadically – there being no definitive form of inheritance.

CHARACTERISTICS

There have been some cases of Smith–Magenis syndrome diagnosed soon after birth, within the first few months of life. Many are not diagnosed, however, until later in childhood when the typical features and behaviour patterns become evident.

Certain features give clues as to the diagnosis:

Certain **facial features** are found in most children with this condition. A smaller than usual **head circumference**, occasionally being microcephalic, is common. The middle part of the rather broad face is flattened, and the nose is small in contrast to the prominent forehead. **Ears**, too, can be an unusual shape and set low on the head.

Short stature is usual, with delayed growth occurring in the early years of life. Later in childhood excessive gain in weight can be a problem. (Due to this feature, this syndrome can be confused with Prader–Willi syndrome, where short stature and excessive weight gain are features. In the Smith–Magenis syndrome, however, the insatiable appetite found in Prader–Willi children is not seen.)

A high proportion of children (around 80%) will be **hyperactive**, and show **self-destructive** and **aggressive** tendencies. These self-destructive aspects include such worrying activities as the child severely injuring the tongue and/or lips by continual chewing. Also, biting – both themselves and other people – is a particular aspects of this condition. There would seem to be a relative insensitivity to pain which may partially account for this type of behaviour.

Along with the general hyperactivity will go **sleep disturbance**, the whole family being exhausted, whilst the child never seems to tire.

Developmental delay is a further feature frequently found in children with the Smith–Magenis syndrome. Learning disability varies from moderate to severe. This feature, when combined with hyperactivity and behaviour problems, causes grave difficulties in management.

Speech delay is a further common problem. This can, of course, be related to the degree of learning disability, but does also seem to be a feature specifically found in children with this syndrome.

Physically, children with the Smith–Magenis syndrome occasionally suffer from **seizures**. Also, **congenital heart defects** are sometimes found. There does also seem to be a higher proportion than usual of middle ear infections in later childhood.

MANAGEMENT IMPLICATIONS

The most difficult aspect in the care of the child with the Smith–Magenis syndrome is the control of the aggressive and self-mutilating **behaviour**. Specialized help from a clinical psychologist for behaviour modification techniques will be of immense help.

Routine **developmental checks** on all aspects of physical and mental development are necessary to determine the level of any retardation that may be present. When the child's abilities are known and school days approach, close liaison between educational and health authorities are vital to determine the best education provision for each individual child.

Repeated **ear infections**, if they occur, must be treated quickly and adequately. Checks on hearing should also be done after each attack of severe otitis. The child with this unpleasant syndrome can do without deafness to compound the problems.

Speech therapy can be helpful, but the degree of learning disability must be borne in mind by therapists when treating these children.

Dietetic advice on **weight control** can also be valuable to avoid the potential long-term problems – and short-term discomfort – of being overweight.

Parents and other family members will need **respite care** at regular intervals. Coping with a hyperactive, and possibly aggressive, child who seems to need practically no sleep can be utterly exhausting.

Genetic counselling, with antenatal screening, if there has already been one affected child in the family, is necessary before further pregnancy.

THE FUTURE

An independent life will never be possible for the child with the Smith–Magenis syndrome. Full-time care will regretfully be necessary for those children and adults with the most severe retardation and difficult behaviour patterns.

Life expectancy does not appear to be reduced – one patient being diagnosed aged 65 years!

SELF-HELP GROUP

Smith–Magenis Support Group
52 Ladeside Close
Newton Mearns
Glasgow G77 6TZ
(Tel. 0141 639 9615)

Aims and provisions: support for families by letter and telephone; information on condition by leaflets; newsletter.

Soto's syndrome

ALTERNATIVE NAME

Cerebral gigantism.

INCIDENCE

Soto's syndrome is a rare genetic growth disorder, the true incidence of which is not recorded, but 150 cases have been reported since 1964. Boys and girls are equally affected.

HISTORY

In 1972 Dr Jaeken reviewed 80 children with the collection of characteristics which make up Soto's syndrome.

CAUSATION

Soto's syndrome is thought to be genetically determined. An autosomal dominant pattern is probable, as evidenced by some families having more than one member with the condition. Otherwise, inheritance is sporadic due to new mutation.

The underlying cause is thought to be a non-progressive abnormality in the hypothalamic region of the brain.

CHARACTERISTICS

Early rapid **growth** is the most obvious and consistent feature of Soto's syndrome. At birth Soto's syndrome babies are usually well up over the 90th centile for length. Growth is rapid throughout the first four or five years of life. Following this time, growth slows, but still persists along the upper ranges of normal. Final adult height is similarly in the upper ranges of normality, with only a very few exceptionally tall adults being recorded.

The **bone age** in children with Soto's syndrome is also advanced.

Tooth eruption and development is also advanced in line with the other bony characteristics.

Facial features: children with Soto's syndrome have a large head with a particularly prominent forehead. Eyes are downward slanting and are set wide apart. The chin is large and a high arched palate is also a feature.

Limbs: hands and feet in Soto's syndrome are also disproportionately large. The arm span frequently can be greater than the child's height!

Learning disability: although by no means invariable, between 50% and 80% (according to different authorities) of Soto's syndrome children have some degree of learning disability. This is generally only mild, but some children are severely disabled.

Other more variable characteristics include the following.

Seizures occasionally occur in this syndrome.

Renal tumours (especially Wilm's tumour) have been reported to have a higher incidence than normal in children with Soto's syndrome.

Clumsiness is evident in many children with this syndrome. This may be part of the underlying cause of the condition, but could be due merely to the rapid growth which occurs during the early years.

MANAGEMENT IMPLICATIONS

Tall stature can cause problems in the pre-school years. Children with Soto's syndrome are both larger and stronger than their peers and have not, as yet, learned how to control their strength and their actions. Hence, care must be taken that these children do not intimidate their playfellows. This can be especially difficult if there is also a degree of learning disability. Strict supervision in playground activities, and guidance in suitable forms of self-expression will be needed.

Suitable clothing and footwear can sometimes be a problem in the three to four year old child. He/she will require sizes more usually recommended for a ten year old child.

Similarly, care must be taken not to expect too much, by way of ability or behaviour, from a child with Soto's syndrome. His/her size can belie the developmental stage attained.

Learning disability: as part of routine developmental screening any persistently low scores in a variety of abilities in relation to age in a large child should alert carers to a possible associated learning problem. Full assessment of abilities in all areas of development will be necessary to determine suitable and appropriate schooling. Children with Soto's syndrome may need education for pupils with moderate learning difficulties, whilst others manage quite adequately in normal educational establishments.

Seizures, although not a common finding in this condition, will need to be investigated in order that appropriate anti-convulsants can be prescribed.

Wilm's tumour: the higher probability of this renal tumour occurring in a child with Soto's syndrome must be remembered. Most frequently the first sign is an abdominal swelling with no other symptoms. Occasionally pain, or blood in the urine, are associated. Surgery, followed by chemotherapy and/or radiotherapy, is the necessary treatment.

THE FUTURE

Children with Soto's syndrome have a normal lifespan with few complications. As mentioned, Wilm's tumours must be remembered during childhood.

During both childhood and adult life, hypo- or hyper-thyroidism is a possibility that must not be overlooked. Appropriate treatment for the condition must then be given.

SELF-HELP GROUP

Soto's Group
73 Parc Castel-y-Mynach
Creigiau
Mid Glamorgan CF4 8NZ
(Tel. 01222 891915)

Aims and provisions: advice and help for parents via telephone and meetings; commissions research; in contact with USA Soto's Group.

Spinal muscular atrophy

ALTERNATIVE NAMES

Werdnig Hoffman disease; Kugelberg–Welander disease.

INCIDENCE

Classification of the varying types of spinal muscular atrophy is somewhat confused as there are a number of different types. Werdnig Hoffman disease (infantile type or type 1) and Kugelberg–Welander (juvenile type or type 3) are the two most common types seen in childhood. (Type 2 is intermediate in severity between the two.)

As the names imply, signs and symptoms of Werdnig Hoffman disease are seen early in life, whilst symptoms of Kugelberg–Welander disease are usually only seen after the age of two years.

The incidence of Werdnig Hoffman disease is reported to be around one in every 25 000 in the north east of England with a slightly lower incidence in this part of the country for the juvenile form – Kugelberg–Welander disease.

There would seem to be a slightly higher incidence in boys than in girls for spinal muscular atrophy diseases. The severity of the juvenile form is less in affected boys.

Chorionic villus sampling is available for antenatal diagnosis.

CAUSATION

Most cases of spinal muscular atrophy appear to be inherited as an autosomal recessive characteristic, but some cases of the juvenile type are inherited as an autosomal dominant.

The basic pathology of all types of spinal muscular atrophy is a degeneration (due to an, as yet, unknown cause) of a particular part of the spinal cord (the anterior horn cells). Following on from this, changes are seen in the muscles controlled by the nerves arising from the affected part of the spinal cord.

CHARACTERISTICS

Werdnig Hoffman disease is the most severe of the three types of spinal muscular atrophy. It is often obvious at birth, when the baby will be extremely **floppy**. Suspicions that there may be something wrong with the baby can often be voiced by the mother when she says that the baby does not seem to be making many movements antenatally. If the condition is not immediately obvious at birth, by three months of age the baby will show definite signs of the disease.

A striking feature of the disease is the difference seen in the movements below the baby's neck from the expressive, alert movements on the face. The main part of the baby's body will be weak and will eventually become paralysed.

A further feature is the rapid, fluttery type of movements (fasciculation) seen in some groups of muscles.

Regretfully, this severe type of spinal muscular atrophy is rapidly progressive with **paralysis** of all muscles, including those around the chest which are intimately concerned with respiration. Death, due to respiratory failure, occurs usually sometime after six months of age and always before the age of three years.

Kugelberg–Welander disease (type 3) differs from the type 1 variety in that signs and symptoms are not seen until after two years of age – and may even be as late as the adolescent years in appearing. The children will be able to learn to walk, although as the disease progresses they will be noticed to have a waddling gait.

The child with this condition will also have difficulty in climbing stairs, and will also find problems in getting back on their feet again after a fall (cf Duchenne muscular dystrophy, which can be confused with Kugelberg–Welander disease in the early stages of the disease).

The disease appears to progress in jumps and starts, often with long periods of time when no further problems are encountered.

Often a **tremor** when the arms are outstretched can be noticed as the disease progresses to involve the arms and shoulder girdle.

Scoliosis (a sideways twist to the spine) can also be a feature.

Intellectual development is normal.

(The type 2 spinal muscular atrophy is intermediate in severity between types 1 and 3. The child is able to sit up unsupported, but cannot stand or walk. Again, the weakness of the muscles is a very obvious sign and there is wasting of the muscles together with a loss of sub-cutaneous fat, so that the child is thin and underweight.

Scoliosis and rib deformities due to the enforced inactivity can give rise to respiratory problems. Many children die, due to this cause, before the age of ten.

INVESTIGATIONS

Electromyogram shows a definitive pattern of disorganized muscle activity.

Biopsy of muscles will show specific changes in these tissues which enable a firm diagnosis to be made.

A specific **enzyme deficiency** has been found in some sufferers from this group of conditions. Maybe it will be found that this condition is yet again a metabolic one, due to a deficiency, or absence, of a vital enzyme.

MANAGEMENT IMPLICATIONS

For the baby with Werdnig Hoffman disease, only normal routine care and nursing is possible. Extra care must be taken to prevent pressure sores arising from paralysed limbs.

Parents must receive practical and emotional help with their disabled baby. The nature of the disease, together with the inevitable outcome, must be sensitively discussed on an on-going basis. It is difficult indeed for parents to come to terms with the fact that their baby will have only a short life, and there will be many questions to be answered as the weeks go by.

Bereavement counselling is also of importance following the death of the child. **Genetic counselling** is advisable when a further pregnancy is envisaged.

The child with Kugelberg–Welander disease will also need much help and routine care as the disease progresses. Routine **developmental checks** will determine the rate of development of motor skills, such as walking, climbing stairs and other activities.

Help, according to the degree of disability, will probably be needed with walking. Physiotherapy skills are extremely valuable in this context. Possible bathing and toileting problems may be encountered – for example, it may be necessary to provide downstairs facilities if climbing stairs is a particular problem.

When school days arrive, teachers must be made aware of their pupil's problems. Pursuit of many physical activities will not be possible. As compensation for this the child should be encouraged to take an interest in more sedentary hobbies and possible later career choices as much as possible.

Special toileting facilities may also need to be made available at school, again depending on the degree of disability. Stairs between classes can also cause difficulties.

Careers must be carefully chosen, and the child with spinal muscular atrophy will need to be encouraged to take an interest in those aspects of work that can be undertaken within the limits of the disease.

THE FUTURE

Life expectancy for people with Kugelberg–Welander disease is near normal.

SELF-HELP GROUP

Jennifer Trust for Spinal Muscular Atrophy
11 Ash Tree Close
Wellesbourne
Warwickshire CV35 9SA
(Tel. 01789 842377)

Aims and provisions: support for affected families; help with provision of aids; leaflets on the condition; newsletter.

Stickler syndrome

ALTERNATIVE NAME

Hereditary progressive arthro-ophthalmopathy.

INCIDENCE

This syndrome is thought to affect one baby in every 20 000 live births. Both sexes can be affected equally. Antenatally, ultra-sonic scan can detect the cleft palate which is a feature in some babies with Stickler syndrome.

The condition can be recognized soon after birth if the 'Robin anomaly' (see below) is present. A positive family history of the condition can also help in making the diagnosis.

HISTORY

Stickler syndrome has some features similar to those seen in the Marfan syndrome – the eye and joint problems being somewhat similar. It has been suggested that Abraham Lincoln and his son, Tad, were both affected by Stickler syndrome, although some historical records show features more like that of Marfan syndrome.

CAUSATION

Stickler syndrome is inherited in an autosomal dominant manner. The affected gene has been mapped to chromosome 12. Not every baby/adult with this syndrome will necessarily show all the features of the condition to the same extent; the expressibility being very variable.

CHARACTERISTICS

Eyes: One of the most constant features of Stickler syndrome is myopia (short-sight). This can be severe from an early age. As is the case for all myopic people (from whatever cause), retinal detachment is an ever-present risk. Up to half of all children with this syndrome will have a complete retinal detachment at some time during their lives – usually during the first 20 years of life. (A retinal detachment is when the retina peels off from the underlying structures. Unless swift diagnosis and treatment is undertaken the result will be permanent blindness.) Marfan's syndrome also has myopia as a characteristic and retinal detachment can also occur as a result. The dislocation of the lens of the eye seen in Marfan's syndrome is, however, not a feature of Stickler syndrome.

Early cataract formation can also occur as part of Stickler syndrome, together with possible glaucoma.

Children with Stickler syndrome can have hypermobile **joints** (cf Marfan's syndrome), but more frequently joints become stiff and at times reddened and enlarged. The joints most commonly affected are ankles, knees and wrists. Occasionally, the joint features may be recognizable at birth. Due to the possible swelling of the joints, locking can be a problem following physical exercise.

Stature: Some children with Stickler syndrome can be tall and thin. Others, however, can be of a normal height and of a rather stocky build.

Facial features can be unusual in some children with this syndrome. The bridge of the nose can be flattened, this feature being more frequently found in children with short stature. In conjunction with the flattened features of the mid-face, a cleft palate can also be present. The lower jaw can also be small and give rise to feeding and breathing difficulties in the early days of life (cf Pierre–Robin syndrome). These two latter features are frequently referred to as the 'Robin anomaly'.

A sensori-neural **hearing loss** occurs with a greater frequency than normal.

MANAGEMENT IMPLICATIONS

In the early days of life, the underdeveloped lower jaw can present feeding difficulties. Feeding the baby in the upright position may be all that is necessary. Breathing can also be obstructed by the baby's tongue falling into the back of the throat due to the smallness of the lower jaw. These babies should be nursed on their sides in the semi-prone position so that the tongue falls forward away from the throat. Ready access to intubation facilities will be necessary if the Robin anomaly is severe.

Surgical repair of the **cleft palate** will need to be done in the early months of life.

The most important feature to be monitored throughout life is the **visual** problem. Myopia must be assessed and corrected with spectacles. Loss, or blurring, of vision must also be urgently investigated so that retinal detachment is diagnosed at an early stage. With early adequate treatment, vision can be saved.

Glaucoma must also be diagnosed and treated in order to preserve vision. (Signs and symptoms of glaucoma include pain in the affected eye, blurring of vision and complaints of seeing 'green haloes' around light sources.)

Possible cataract formation will need to be routinely checked and appropriate action taken where necessary.

The possible hypermobility of **joints** and periods of reddening and swelling will mean that violent physical exercise should be avoided by children with Stickler syndrome. Contact sports of all kinds, in particular, should not be allowed. Episodes of painful red and swollen joints will need appropriate periods of rest and pain relief. The help of a physiotherapist is valuable following these episodes.

Schooling will depend on the degree of visual problems present. Special facilities will be necessary for those children with the most severe visual or hearing loss. Careers which depend on good vision or hearing are not suitable.

Children with Stickler syndrome have no loss of intellectual ability.

THE FUTURE

Severe visual loss is the most serious and disabling of the features that can occur with this syndrome. It is thought that all children will have some definite visual abnormalities by the age of ten years.

With care and gentle graded exercises, joint mobility can be maintained throughout life, although osteo-arthritis can develop later in life.

Severe deafness may become an added burden later.

SELF-HELP GROUP

Stickler Syndrome Support Group
c/o Contact-a-Family
170 Tottenham Court Road
London W1P 0HA
(Tel. 0171 383 3555)

Aims and provisions: information on the syndrome; support for affected families.

Sturge–Weber syndrome

INCIDENCE

The number of people with this unusual syndrome is unknown, but it is thought to be a rare condition. Both sexes are affected equally.

CAUSATION

The reasons behind the occurrence of the Sturge-Weber syndrome are unknown. There does not seem, at present, to be any evidence that it is an inherited disorder. The most probable cause is a new mutation occurring sporadically.

There is no antenatal diagnosis available, but the typical signs on the baby's face are obvious at birth.

CHARACTERISTICS

A **'port-wine'** stain on one half of the baby's face is the very noticeable characteristic seen at birth. This specialized type of 'birthmark' follows the course of the fifth cranial nerve. This particular nerve is divided into three branches, supplying the forehead, cheek region and lower jaw respectively. The upper branch is most often affected in the Sturge–Weber syndrome, but all three branches can be affected so that the whole side of the face is covered by the purplish mark. The basic cause of this lies in an abnormality in the walls of the tiny blood vessels supplying the skin.

Parts of the blood supply to the **brain** may also be affected. On X-ray, specific 'tram-line' areas of calcification can be seen to appear when the child is over the age of two years.

Seizures are often a complication of this syndrome. The usual age of onset of these is after one to two years of age. This fits in with the altered X-ray appearance in the brain round about this age.

Sometimes **paralysis** of one half of the body occurs.

Both these latter characteristics are also due to the basic abnormality in the walls of the blood vessels which causes the naevus on the baby's face.

Eyes: At times, **glaucoma** can occur in the eye on the same side as the port-wine stain. The narrow passage which allows the fluid inside the eye to drain becomes blocked by the blood vessel abnormality, causing tension inside the eyeball to increase dangerously. This condition, if not treated, can lead to blindness in the affected eye. Occasionally, the colour of the eyes may differ from each other. The eye on the affected side can be blue, even though the other eye is brown. This again is due to the abnormality affecting the blood vessels at the back of the eye.

MANAGEMENT IMPLICATIONS

Port-wine stain: There is no easy treatment for this type of birthmark, particularly if it occupies an extensive area. Laser treatment is available in some centres, but this is time-consuming as only small areas can be done at any one time. Expense is also a problem. Cosmetic cover-up creams are available which give very good results at obscuring the mark, but these are more likely to be used later in life rather than in childhood.

Seizures will need to be treated with anti-convulsant drugs, and several may need to be tried before the right one, or combination of drugs, is found to be effective. If the fits cannot be controlled by medication, surgery to specific affected areas of the brain can be of value.

Glaucoma needs urgent treatment by eyedrops or surgery. Without treatment, blindness can result.

Emotional problems can occur, especially in the teenage years, and also particularly in girls. Teasing about the facial disfigurement can lead children to become withdrawn. The help of a clinical psychologist will be valuable in the most severely affected children.

THE FUTURE

This will very much depend on the extent, and sites, of the abnormalities in the walls of the blood vessels. If only the skin of the face is involved there is no threat to life or health, but if the disease is more extensive and affects other blood vessels in the brain, seizures can be a grave problem with potentially fatal results.

SELF-HELP GROUP

Sturge–Weber Foundation (UK)
53 Brookland road West
Old Swan
Liverpool L13 2BG
(Tel. 0151 220 5290)

Aims and provisions: support, advice and information for affected families; promotes medical research.

TAR syndrome

ALTERNATIVE NAME

Absent radius-thrombocytopaenia.

INCIDENCE

This is a relatively rare syndrome, but over 100 cases have been reported in the literature. There appears to be no special geographical location, or ethnic groups in which there are a greater number of cases.

There would appear to be more girls affected than boys. The reason for this is thought to be that boys may be so severely affected by the condition that death occurs *in utero*. Ultra-sound examination during pregnancy – from 18 weeks onward – can detect the specific abnormality in the baby's arms.

HISTORY

The common name of this syndrome is an acronym on the abnormalities found – **T**hrombocytopaenia, **A**bsent **R**adius.

CAUSATION

This syndrome is inherited in an autosomal recessive manner.

CHARACTERISTICS

Blood system

Thrombocytopaenia – a reduction in the number of platelets circulating in the blood – is one of the main features of this syndrome. (Platelets play a vital role in the normal clotting of blood.) As well as the reduced numbers of platelets circulating in the blood, there are also abnormalities in the function of those that are present in the most severe cases.

This feature will result in abnormal **bleeding** in various parts of the body – for example, bleeding from the bowel or nose and excessive bruising from very minor injuries.

Over 90% of new-born babies with this condition will suffer from some episode of bleeding during their first few months of life. This bleeding can be severe and life-threatening, and it is thought that around 30% of babies with this syndrome die before one year of age due to uncontrollable bleeding.

If the first few critical months are survived, the episodes of bleeding tend to occur in a more episodic fashion related to some form of bodily stress; for example, an infection or a necessary surgical operation. Also, even in the most severely affected baby, the platelet count will tend to improve as the years go by – so that, once again, the episodes of severe bleeding will tend to occur only with stressful events, as outlined above.

Anaemia can be an ever-present concern, due to the blood loss through the frequent bleeding episodes and also possibly due to other blood abnormalities.

Skeletal system

The other main feature of the TAR syndrome is the absence of the **radius** from the child's forearm. (The radius is one of the two long bones linking the elbow to the wrist.) Usually both arms are affected by this abnormality.

In some children there are also abnormalities of the bones of the **hands**. As well as this possible bony abnormality, further deformities can occur in the hands due to the unequal and unusual pull of the muscles which normally act on the radius, but which now act on the bones of the wrist. Children with this deformity will – understandably – be slower than their peers in gaining manual dexterity. Eventually, however, motor function is good, with help and practice.

Other problems can also occur in different parts of the skeleton. For example, **hips** can be dislocated, **knees** stiff with occasional dislocation of the knee cap, or **ribs** and **spine** can show abnormalities. These latter abnormalities can cause the child to have a **short stature**.

These skeletal features will vary from child to child.

The blood and skeletal characteristics are always found in children with the TAR syndrome, but the following features can also occur:

- **Heart defects** of various types can be present. Fallot's tetralogy (in which there are four specific heart abnormalities) or an atrial septal defect (or 'hole' between the two upper chambers of the heart) are the most commonly found.
- **Learning disability** can very occasionally occur if there has been bleeding into the brain at an early stage in life.
- **Allergy** to cow's milk has been reported in an above average number of children with the TAR syndrome.

MANAGEMENT IMPLICATIONS

Blood: Each episode of bleeding must be treated with urgency. This is of especial importance in the early days of life when these events are more common. Transfusion of either whole blood or platelets may be necessary with a severe bleed.

As the baby matures and begins to crawl and walk, the inevitable **minor injuries** must be reduced to a minimum as far as possible. Again, urgent medical treatment must be sought if serious bleeding occurs.

It is also important to avoid **infections** as far as is possible without over-protecting the child too much. Each bout of infection should be treated aggressively in order to reduce the risk of bleeding due to the abnormal clotting mechanism found in the TAR syndrome.

Anaemia should also be checked for whenever a child appears listless, without energy or looks especially pale. This will, of course, be particularly important after an episode of bleeding.

Skeletal: The advice of an orthopaedic surgeon can be valuable. Possible realigning of muscles in the arm to improve function may be necessary.

Physiotherapy help, in the early days, when hand and arm dexterity are being learned, is valuable. Orthopaedic appliances, in the form of braces, can be helpful, and should be fitted early for maximum effect.

Possible **heart defects** will need to be assessed and treatment decided upon by a paediatric cardiologist.

Schooling will need to be geared to the child's individual physical abilities. (Intellectual ability is generally normal, unless intra-cranial haemorrhage in the very early days of life has left irreparable brain damage.) Children with the TAR syndrome will need extra help with writing and drawing skills. Typewriters and/or word-processors can be an option at a later date.

Contact sports should be avoided, due to the ever-present possibility of bleeding from even minor trauma.

Careers will need careful consideration due both to the physical and bleeding problems.

Any **cow's milk allergy** will need dietary advice with an alternative milk supply – goat's milk or soy milk, for example.

THE FUTURE

Outlook for life expectancy is good once the difficult, and potentially fatal, days of early childhood are successfully passed.

Women will tend to suffer from heavy menstrual periods, and watch must be kept for anaemia due to this.

SELF-HELP GROUP

TAR Syndrome Support Group
13 Friarside
Witton Gilbert
Durham DH7 6RY
(Tel. 0191 371 0055)

Aims and provisions: information about the condition; support for affected families; newsletter.

Tay–Sachs disease

ALTERNATIVE NAME

GM2 gangliosidosis.

INCIDENCE

This condition is usually only seen in Ashkenazi Jewish families, where the incidence is thought to be as high as around one in every 4000 live births. A further population group in which this serious condition occurs is French Canadians. Older children and adults are virtually never seen with Tay–Sachs disease, as death inevitably occurs in early childhood.

Boys and girls can be equally affected.

CAUSATION

Tay–Sachs disease is inherited as an autosomal recessive. There are large numbers of people in the particular population groups mentioned above that carry the abnormal gene; the figure is thought to be as high as one in every 25 people. So, in spite of early death, there is still a great reservoir of people carrying this serious condition. Tay–Sachs disease is a further example of a condition which arises due to a specific enzyme defect. This deficiency allows certain chemical substances to build up in various parts of the body. These then give rise to the specific characteristics of the disease. The enzyme involved in this case is hexosaminidase A. The substance which is not adequately metabolized, due to lack of this enzyme, is a ganglioside.

Antenatal diagnosis is available by chorionic villus sampling.

CHARACTERISTICS

Tay–Sachs disease can be divided into two types, according to when the typical signs and symptoms make their appearance. In the 'infantile' type, the characteristic features begin to appear within the first six months of life. The 'late infantile' type (also known as Sandhoff's disease) will not show any sign of the typical features until the child is around two to three years of age. In this latter type two enzymes are involved – hexosaminidase A and B. In both types the features are the same, only the timing being different. All features are due to an abnormal storage in various parts of the body, but particularly in the grey matter of the brain, of the GM2 ganglioside.

Vision: In the infantile type of Tay–Sachs disease the baby of around six months of age will begin to disregard movements around him/her which had previously attracted his/her attention. An increased 'startle' response will be seen so that, for example, a person who has been nearby for some time will suddenly make him/her jump. Part of the reason for this increased 'startle' reaction may be, in addition to failing vision, a **hypersensitivity to sound**. This feature is one of the earliest signs that the disease may be present. On ophthalmic examination, a cherry red spot on a particular part of the retina will be visible. This is a direct result of the build-up of ganglioside in this part of the eye. Within a very short time, the baby's vision will deteriorate so much that he/she will be quite blind, usually by one year of age.

Developmentally, loss of skills already learned is also an early sign of Tay–Sachs disease. The baby who will have been gurgling, smiling, lifting his/her head and moving arms and legs vigorously will become limp and unresponsive. This can be devastating to the parents who have been watching with delight their baby's increasing awareness of his/her surroundings. As with all the metabolic conditions, the deterioration of a seemingly normal baby can be almost unbelievable.

Seizures commonly begin to occur during the second year of life. Often, they will take the form of outbursts of quite inappropriate laughter. The EEG will show abnormalities in association with this event. These fits can be very difficult to control, and a number of anti-convulsant drugs may need to be tried before some degree of control is gained. As the disease progresses the episodes of seizures tends to lessen spontaneously.

Hypotonia, or a generalized weakness of all the muscles, rapidly follows. The baby who previously had been rolling over and attempting to pull his/her head and shoulders into a sitting position will cease to try this. He/she will lie apathetically in his/her cot becoming more and more unresponsive to his/her surroundings. Only sudden loud noises will cause a 'startle' reaction along with the outbursts of laughter which denote a fit.

Eventually the baby's limbs will become stiff with exaggerated reflexes until a complete spastic paralysis results.

Head size can increase rapidly due to the deposition of abnormal material in the brain. This can give the appearance of hydrocephalus, although this is not the true cause of the increase in head circumference. (Hydrocephalus implies an increase in size of the ventricles in the brain containing cerebrospinal fluid.)

The final outcome of this tragic decease is death by the age of three to four years. In the late infantile type (Sandhoff's disease) the characteristic features do not begin to make their appearance before two to three years of age, but a similar rapid deterioration as seen in the infantile type proceeds and death usually occurs between the ages of five and ten years.

MANAGEMENT IMPLICATIONS

Support for, and explanation to, the parents is a vital part of this tragic genetic condition. Parents will need to have explanations as to the inheritance of their baby's illness, the cause of the disease and the expected age of the final outcome.

Appropriate nursing care, together with help for parents on this aspect as long as it is possible for the child to be cared for at home, is virtually all that can be done. Eventually, full-time nursing care will be a necessity. Respite care, whilst the baby remains at home, so that parents and any other members of the family can have a holiday without the continuous worry of caring for a very disabled child, is important.

Genetic counselling for couples considering a further pregnancy is advisable so that the risks of having a further child with the condition can be estimated.

SELF-HELP GROUP

Tay–Sachs and Allied Diseases Association
Golden Gates Lodge
Weston Road
Crewe
Cheshire CW1 1XN
(Tel. 01270 250221)

Aims and provisions: support for parents; promotes research; publications and information on screening. (This is a branch of the Research Trust in Metabolic Disease in Children, also at this address.)

Thalassaemia

ALTERNATIVE NAMES

Cooley anaemia; mediterranean anaemia.

INCIDENCE

As with sickle cell anaemia, thalassaemia is a haemaglobinopathy, and only occurs in certain racial groups – mainly in tropical and sub-tropical parts of Europe, Africa and Asia.

As the alternative name, mediterranean anaemia, implies, there is a high incidence around the Mediterranean Sea; the disease being virtually unknown amongst Northern European races. The incidence is variable, but amongst some populations, it can be as high as one in every 100 births.

Twenty per cent of the populations of Turkey and Greece are thought to suffer from the disease. There is also a high incidence in Burma and Thailand.

Both sexes are equally affected.

Antenatal diagnosis by chorionic villus sampling at ten weeks of pregnancy and/or foetal blood sampling at 20 weeks of pregnancy is possible.

(It is important that thalassaemia major (which is discussed here) is definitively differentiated from the milder form, thalassaemia intermedia, as the course of the disease and also the treatment differ.)

HISTORY

The name thalassaemia was deduced from 'thallus', meaning an 'inland sea', the Mediterranean.

CAUSATION

Thalassaemia is inherited as an autosomal recessive condition. The basic abnormality is one of deficient production of haemoglobin – the oxygen-carrying part of the blood found in the red blood cells. One of the specific globulins necessary for the proper metabolism of haemoglobin is not synthesised adequately, leading to anaemia.

There are two main types of thalassaemia – alpha and beta – with a number of complicated variants of both types. A particularly severe form of alpha thalassaemia results in still-birth or death of the affected baby within a few hours of birth.

CHARACTERISTICS (BETA THALASSAEMIA)

The baby with thalassaemia is usually fit and well at birth, but by three to six months of age will show signs of:

- **Anaemia**: The baby will become pale and listless, unwilling to take feeds and may vomit what little food is taken.
- **Jaundice** may also be present from an early stage. This yellow coloration of the skin and mucous membranes is caused by the more rapid than usual breakdown of the red blood cells.

Enlargement of the **liver** and **spleen** are also specific features associated with thalassaemia. These characteristics are due to:

- the body attempting to produce red blood cells in parts of the body other than the bone-marrow;
- changes relating to the anaemia, which by putting an extra load on the heart causes back-pressure on the liver;
- extra deposits of iron-containing substances which, in turn, is a long-term result of the anaemia.

Bones can also eventually become thinned as a result of the body's attempts to produce adequate haemoglobin for daily needs. Ultimately, this can lead to fractures and deformity.

COMPLICATIONS

These are mainly secondary effects due to the excess storage of iron in the body. This is partly due to the disease itself and partly due to the necessity of frequent blood transfusions.

Heart arrhythmias – these can be difficult to control and can be fatal.

Cirrhosis of the liver this may lead to eventual liver failure.

Diabetes – this can also occur, due to failure of the specific cells in the pancreas to produce adequate insulin caused, once again, by the iron overload.

MANAGEMENT IMPLICATIONS

In severe cases of thalassaemia, **frequent blood transfusions** are necessary to combat the persistent anaemia. Specialized control of the type of blood given and the frequency of the transfusions will be necessary to reduce complications to a minimum.

Removal of the spleen (**splenectomy**) may be necessary. Extra care must be taken following this regarding **infections** of all kinds. For example, if a child has a fever for no obvious reason, hospital admission to discover the source of the infection will be needed with a degree of urgency. Parents must be advised to contact the thalassaemia clinic or their own doctor under these circumstances.

Alongside the need for frequent blood transfusions must be special chelating (iron-removing) treatment in an attempt to minimize the amount of iron stored in various parts of the body. This can be done either by a sub-cutaneous infusion with a special 'pump', or by giving the substance together with the blood at the time of transfusion. Vitamin C is also a necessary dietary additive to assist in the removal of iron. (Due to the necessary long-term nature of this chelating process with little obvious effect, parents can at times find it difficult to insist that their child follows these routines. Time spent giving explanations and encouragement is, therefore, a necessary part of the treatment.

It is important that regular checks on development and **growth** of children with thalassaemia are carried out. Height and weight should be plotted serially on a centile chart. Also, in children under the age of 12 years, annual X-rays of the bones of the hand and wrist should be done as a measure of normal bone growth.

Schooling for the child with thalassaemia will need to take into account the probable frequent absences necessary for transfusion purposes. Liaison between home and school, with work sent home when the child is feeling well enough, will ensure that close touch is kept with peers. Teachers should also have a basic understanding of the effects of the disease on their pupils.

Close watch, on a regular basis, will need to be kept for signs of liver, cardiac and endocrine complications of thalassaemia. **Blood** tests to determine liver, pancreatic and thyroid function will need to be performed routinely.

Every person suffering from one of the haemoglobinopathies should have a **haemoglobinopathy card** so that, in case of emergency, medical staff will be aware of the inherited disease and the need for extra care in treatment. (A national card was produced in 1988, but many hospitals have produced their own local version.)

Emotional and practical support both for parents and child are an important part of care. A balance must be kept between over-protection of the child and the need for constant care and treatment. This can be an especially difficult problem during adolescence when the affected child must learn to take control of treatment. The specialized centres for haemoglobinopathy disease can do much to help this transition into adulthood, along with help from the appropriate self help group.

THE FUTURE

For people with severe thalassaemia, life expectancy is shortened, largely due to the effects of the iron overload in various tissues and organs of the body. With the improved methods of chelation, however, the outlook is improving.

Genetic counselling is advisable for families suffering from this inherited disease.

Bone-marrow transplantation – ideally before the age of 12 years when damage by excess iron is less likely – is the treatment currently being explored. Research continues into a chelating agent which can be taken by mouth.

SELF-HELP GROUP

UK Thalassaemia Society
107 Nightingale Lane
London N8 7QY
(Tel. 0181 348 0437)

Aims and provisions: advice, information and support for families; fund-raising for research; information sheets available in Italian, Greek, Turkish, Hindi, Punjabi, Gujerati and Chinese as well as English.

Treacher Collins syndrome

ALTERNATIVE NAMES

Dysostosis mandibulo-facial; Franceschetti–Klein syndrome.

INCIDENCE

The number of people suffering from this syndrome is not known. A number of families with the disease, throughout several generations, have been described and researched.

HISTORY

In 1933, Dr Treacher Collins first described people with the particular characteristics seen in this syndrome, in a paper presented to the Ophthalmology Society of the UK.

CAUSATION

This syndrome is inherited as an autosomal dominant. The penetrance rate appears to be high, but the degree to which sufferers are affected is variable. There is a high rate of mutations accounting for this syndrome and about half of all the cases described are thought to be due to this cause. Some of the babies born with Treacher Collins syndrome, caused by a new mutation, have fathers who are older than normal.

This syndrome has been successfully diagnosed antenatally using fetoscopic methods. The specific characteristics have also been seen on ultrasonic screening.

CHARACTERISTICS

The abnormalities seen in the Treacher Collins syndrome solely affect the face and associated anatomical structures.

The bones of the **cheeks** (maxillae) are small and under-developed. This gives the false impression of a large nose, which is often initially the most noticeable feature.

The **lower jaw** can also be small, giving the appearance of a receding chin. This feature can lead to problems with respiration and feeding during the early days of life. During the relaxation of muscles during sleep, the tiny, under-developed jaw can drop back. This allows the baby's tongue to fall back into his/her throat and effectively obstruct breathing. This is especially dangerous if the baby is put to sleep on his/her back. The safest position for these babies is on their sides (putting babies to sleep on their tummies is thought to be a possible factor in the causation of the sudden infant death syndrome, and so should be avoided, even though it would appear to be an ideal position for the Treacher Collins baby).

Feeding, too, can be difficult due to the small jaw. A good 'seal' around nipple or teat is almost impossible to obtain until the baby matures and his/her lower jaw develops further.

Eyes have a downward slant at the outside edge, compounding the unusual features of the face. The lower **eyelids** may have a small gap, or 'nick' in their length (coloboma), and **eyelashes** may be absent on the nasal side of this feature. Fortunately, this coloboma never seems to affect any other structures of the eye, as is the case in some other syndromes – the CHARGE association, for example. There is no visual defect associated with the Treacher Collins syndrome.

Ears can be small and malformed. The internal parts of the ears, including the external auditory canal and the middle ear can also be abnormally developed. In around half the children with the Treacher Collins syndrome, a conductive deafness occurs as a result of these abnormalities.

Occasionally (in about 28% of cases) the baby with Treacher Collins syndrome may be born with a **cleft palate**. If present, this will add to the early feeding difficulties.

A **heart defect** has also occasionally been found with this syndrome.

Due to the abnormalities possible both in upper and lower jaws, there may be problems with proper eruption of **teeth** at a later date.

MANAGEMENT IMPLICATIONS

Early **breathing** and **feeding** difficulties, if specific abnormalities are severe, will need skilled specialized attention. Nasogastric feeding may be necessary if sucking is impossible in the first few weeks of life. A temporary tracheostomy may be necessary in the most severely affected children.

Surgery may be needed to repair a **cleft palate** if this is present. Surgery may also be necessary to repair some of the unusual facial features. Great improvement is possible with plastic surgery, particularly to the problems in the upper jaw.

The most important aspect of care for the child with the Treacher Collins syndrome is the early diagnosis of any **conductive deafness** that may arise due to the abnormalities in the auditory system. It has been regrettable in the past that children with severe hearing problems have been thought to have learning disabilities, with the result that both educational facilities and general handling have been inappropriate. Hearing aids may be necessary from an early age, and this help with hearing will ensure that development is not delayed in other fields.

Orthodontic help may be required later on in childhood if teeth erupt crookedly.

Emotional support, especially if teasing at school occurs due to the child's unusual facial features, may be necessary for both child and parents from professionals concerned with the welfare of the family.

THE FUTURE

Life expectancy is normal. A normal career choice is open to the child with Treacher Collins syndrome with the exception of deafness being a possible limiting factor for some careers.

Genetic counselling is advisable before pregnancy is embarked upon.

SELF-HELP GROUPS

Treacher Collins Support Group
114 Vincent Road
Thorpe Hamlet
Norwich
Norfolk NR1 4HH
(Tel. 01603 33736)

Aims and provisions: support and friendship for sufferers and their families; information by newsletter and reports on the syndrome.

A special group, dealing with all cases of facial disfigurement, is also helpful for families with a child with the Treacher Collins syndrome:

'Let's Face It' (network for the facially disfigured)
10 Wood End
Crowthorne
Berkshire RG11 6DQ
(Tel. 01344 774405)

Tuberous sclerosis

INCIDENCE

The estimated incidence of tuberous sclerosis is between one in every 30 000 to 40 000 live births. It is of importance as it is thought to account for 0.5% of all children with a significant learning disability. Both boys and girls are affected equally.

HISTORY

Tuberous sclerosis was first recognized in 1880 by a Dr Bournville, who described the pathological changes in the brain. In 1908 Dr Vogt put the triad of features together – learning disability, convulsions and the specific type of rash. In 1969, the genetic causation of the condition was described.

Much interest and work, particularly in the USA, has taken place over the past 20 years. This has resulted in further understanding of the possible long-term effects of the condition.

The name, tuberous sclerosis, is derived form the tuber-like swellings which occur and harden (sclerosis) in various tissues and organs of the body.

CAUSATION

Tuberous sclerosis can be dominantly inherited, but many cases are the result of new mutations. Widely differing degrees of severity occur. In 1987, there was evidence that the gene for tuberous sclerosis is situated on chromosome 9.

There is no known antenatal diagnosis at present. But if one or other of the parents is known to have the condition, ultra-sonic scanning can detect tumours in the baby's heart as early as the 20th week of pregnancy.

CHARACTERISTICS

Infantile spasms may be the first sign to alert to a diagnosis of tuberous sclerosis. These are a very specific type of convulsions occurring in early infancy, in which the baby bends at the hips a number of times in very rapid succession. (These attacks are also known as 'salaam' attacks.) A characteristic pattern is seen on EEG. Affected children can suffer from fits throughout life.

Skin lesions of a specific nature may be the first sign if convulsions do not occur in infancy.

Areas of **lesser pigmentation** than the surrounding skin may occur often characteristically in the shape of an ash leaf. '**Shagreen patches**' also appear, particularly over the lower back. These patches are areas of raised, thickened, slightly pigmented skin.

Later in childhood, the typical '**adenoma sebaceum**' appear round the nose and in a butterfly shape across the cheeks. They can extend to the forehead and chin, but rarely extend below the neck. In spite of the name, these lesions are nothing to do with the sebaceous glands, but are naevi surrounding the hair follicles.

Cafe-au-lait spots, similar to those seen in neurofibromatosis, can also occur, although not in such large numbers. (Tuberous sclerosis is not connected with neurofibromatosis in any way apart from this aspect).

Tumours of varying size and type are also found in various organs of the body, such as the heart, brain, liver, spleen and kidneys, in addition to being found in the bones. These will not all occur in any one individual with tuberous sclerosis, but the possibility of this occurring must be uppermost when symptoms relating to various bodily systems arise.

Teeth: pitting is often seen in the enamel of the teeth, and fibrous growths can also occur in the gums.

Learning disability is found in just over half of the children with tuberous sclerosis. The learning disability is usually obvious by the time the child is two years old. The remaining children have normal intelligence.

Children with learning disability due to tuberous sclerosis can also exhibit behaviour problems. These take the form of outbursts of rage and other inappropriate manifestations. When the child reaches the teenage years, these can be even more difficult to control due to size and physical abilities.

Varying degrees of tuberous sclerosis can occur – for example, only the skin lesions may be visible in a parent of a child with tuberous sclerosis. Silent tumours could be present in the brain or other parts of the body under these circumstances. This is of importance in genetic counselling.

MANAGEMENT IMPLICATIONS

Treatment is symptomatic as there is no cure for tuberous sclerosis.

Convulsions: it is important to control early convulsions as far as possible, as this is thought possibly to prevent the onset of learning disability. A CT scan will determine the site of the lesions in the brain – the 'tubers' described by Bournville. (Similarly, parents of children with tuberosis sclerosis who have the typical skin lesions only should be investigated by CT scanning.)

Ultra-sound investigation of heart and kidneys is a sensible precaution to exclude lesions in these organs, particularly if there are any related symptoms.

Follow-up of children with tuberous sclerosis is of importance to diagnose and treat as far as possible any problems relating to potential tumours in various parts of the body.

Learning disability: it is important that assessment of the individual child's abilities is made and reviewed on a regular basis. Schooling must be appropriate to the individual child's needs. Advice both to parents and teachers at each stage is of vital importance. Behaviour problems, if severe, can benefit from the help of a clinical psychologist.

Dental care is important due to the frequent poor state of the enamel.

Genetic counselling of parents considering further children must also be offered, in addition to offering the same counselling to the child with tuberous sclerosis when he/she reaches reproductive age.

THE FUTURE

Half of the children with tuberous sclerosis will lead normal lives, and will only need to be aware of the possibility of manifestations of their condition in a wide variety of organs throughout their body. Other children with tuberous sclerosis who have a varying degree of learning disability will need advice on work prospects, and a few with severe learning disability will need full-time care throughout their lives.

Lifespan is dependent upon the presence, or otherwise, of tumours in various vital organs of the body.

The first of a number of specialist clinics for tuberous sclerosis sufferers was established in 1990. Advice is given on diagnosis, management and genetic counselling.

SELF-HELP GROUP

Tuberous Sclerosis Association of Great Britain
Little Barnsley Farm
Catshill
Bromsgrove
Worcestershire B61 ONQ
(Tel. 01527 871898)

Aims and provisions: practical and emotional support; fact sheet on tuberous sclerosis; research funding.

Turner's syndrome

ALTERNATIVE NAMES

Chromosome 45/X syndrome; Ullrich–Turner syndrome.

INCIDENCE

For approximately every 2500 live female births, one girl will be affected by Turner's syndrome. (Only girls are affected, due to the mode of inheritance.) Sufferers from Turner's syndrome will not necessarily show all the syndrome's features, but there will be sufficient evidence to support a clinical diagnosis of Turner's syndrome.

HISTORY

Turner's syndrome was first defined by Dr Henry Turner in 1938. This American doctor described four of the clinical features – small stature, lack of sexual development, webbed neck and a wide carrying angle at the elbows – in adult women. Later it was found that these women had high levels of gonadotrophins in their urine, together with a complete lack of ovarian tissue. These vital sexual organs are replaced by whorls of connective tissue.

It was not until 1959 that the genetic background to the condition was demonstrated.

CAUSATION

Girls with Turner's syndrome have only 45 chromosomes instead of the usual full complement of 46. The chromosome missing is one of the X chromosomes. (XX denotes a female and XY a male. Turner's syndrome girls are denoted as XO). However, some girls with Turner's syndrome have a 'mosaic' chromosomal pattern, i.e. some cells have the full complement of sex chromosomes. Such chromosome patterns are denoted as XO/XX. This can be reflected in the clinical picture.

As 99% of girls with Turner's syndrome are infertile, there is small chance of the condition being inherited from the female side. The missing chromosome is lost during cell division. In the literature there are 54 reported pregnancies in Turner's syndrome women. The outcome has been variable, over half of the babies being miscarried or still-born. A few pregnancies have resulted in the birth of normal children.

CHARACTERISTICS

Short stature is the most consistent and obvious problem. Growth is usually within normal limits until around three years of age, although the baby may be significantly shorter at birth. After this time, the girl with Turner's syndrome will fall progressively behind her school friends in height. This failure to grow is also very marked during the early teenage years when the normal growth spurt of puberty should occur. Special charts to plot the growth of Turner's syndrome girls are available. Final height will be a maximum of 5 feet (150 cm), but more usually only 4 feet 8 inches (141 cm) is reached. Treatment may assist in increasing height.

Fertility: Due to the non-development of the ovaries, all true Turner's syndrome girls will be unable to conceive. Also as a result of this ovarian problem, puberty can be a difficult time, as secondary sexual characteristics fail to develop without treatment. Breasts do not develop, pubic hair does not appear and menstruation does not occur.

Heart: Girls with Turner's syndrome are more likely than their peers to suffer from co-arctation (narrowing) of the aorta. This means that there may be raised blood pressure and peripheral vascular problems later in life unless treatment is given. Other heart anomalies can also occur.

Eyes: There is a higher incidence than normal of visual problems – either long-sight or short-sight, for which glasses may be necessary. Squint is also more common, and epicanthic folds and drooping eyelids (ptosis) can give a false impression of sleepiness.

Ears: Turner's syndrome girls often suffer frequently from otitis media. This can lead to a conductive deafness if not adequately treated.

Intelligence is usually normal in Turner's syndrome girls, but some may have specific learning difficulties. For example, number concepts and word presentation can pose problems.

Thyroid function: There is a higher incidence than normal of hypothyroidism, due to lymphocytic thyroiditis, in Turner's syndrome.

The following added features may, or may not, be seen.

- **Webbing of the neck** is a fairly common feature, and may be one of the first clues in infancy. Loose folds of skin may also be seen in the nape of the neck in the young baby.
- Swelling of the backs of the **hands** and **feet** is also common during infancy, and is due to faulty lymphatic drainage. This may persist throughout life.
- A **broad chest** with widely spaced nipples is a fairly consistent feature.
- There is a wide carrying angle at the **elbows**.
- **Low-set ears** can also be a feature.
- A **high-arched palate** can occur, with the result that the teeth may be overcrowded.
- A **shortened fourth finger** is seen in 50% of Turner's syndrome girls.

All these latter features are coincidental findings which may, or may not, be present in girls with Turner's syndrome. Few of them cause problems, but, if they are present, they can assist clinical diagnosis.

MANAGEMENT IMPLICATIONS

Nothing can be done medically to alter the **infertile state**, due to the complete lack of ovarian tissue. Much can be done, however, to ensure that **secondary sexual characteristics** develop normally. At puberty, around 12 to 13 years, oestrogen in some form may be given. This will ensure breast development, the growth of pubic hair and the maturation of the uterus to normal size. The vaginal epithelium also matures. When these changes are fully under way, cyclical treatment with the appropriate hormone is started. This will ensure that menstruation occurs regularly, although, of course, without ovulation. This treatment must continue at least until the natural menopausal age.

Short stature: steroids can be given and help in many cases to increase final height, but even with this treatment, final height is never more than 5 feet. This characteristic may present educational problems as schooling progresses. Physical education in particular can often be difficult for these shorter children. Care must be taken not to treat Turner's syndrome children as younger than they really are, due to their lack of height and the lack of secondary sexual characteristics.

Co-arctation of the aorta, if present, must be corrected surgically. This abnormality should be discovered at routine developmental checks when femoral pulses are found to be diminished.

Eyes: continuing checks must be made for refractory errors, and glasses prescribed where necessary. Squints should be corrected, both to prevent amblyopia and for cosmetic purposes.

Ears: Frequent bouts of otitis media should be adequately treated and hearing tested regularly after each severe infection. 'Glue' ear is common and may need myringotomy and insertion of ventilation tubes. School teachers should be made aware of potential problems in this area.

Feeding problems can occur in infancy in Turner's syndrome. The cause of this is not clear, but symptomatic treatment and support will ensure that babies grow through this phase satisfactorily.

Watch must be maintained throughout life for signs of **hypothyroidism** – unusual weight gain, slowness of action and speech, hoarse voice, dry skin and scanty hair. Replacement therapy with thyroxine may be indicated under these conditions.

Specific **learning difficulties** may occur, particularly in word comprehension and presentation. Similarly, there may be difficulties with mathematical concepts. Intelligence is generally normal, but there may be mild learning disability. In the UK, the 'statementing' procedure may be required to ensure that Turner's syndrome children obtain the best possible educational facilities. There may also be **spatial difficulties** with large movements, such as throwing and catching balls. Fine movements, such as used in painting, drawing and sewing are all usually within normal limits. Care should therefore be taken to put emphasis on and give encouragement in these latter tasks, and to avoid upset and frustration with other wide-ranging activities.

THE FUTURE

Turner's syndrome girls can expect a normal lifespan. The greatest sadness is the inability to have children, but in-vitro fertilization by donor ova is possible as the uterus is normal. Adoption and fostering are also possibilities.

Sexual feelings and relationships are normal, as vagina and uterus are of normal size.

Clothes may be a problem, due to the small sizes necessary being of too young a style. Also Turner's syndrome girls do tend to put on weight easily as they get older. This can add to the clothing problem. Home dressmaking is a good option to pursue.

SELF-HELP GROUP

The Turner Syndrome Society
(The Child Growth Foundation)
2 Mayfield Avenue
London W4 1PW
(Tel. 0181 994 7625; 0181 995 0257)

Aims and provisions: to offer advice and help to women and girls with Turner's syndrome; to commission research through the Child Growth Foundation; to raise awareness of the syndrome and to provide counselling.

Usher's syndrome

INCIDENCE

Reports on the incidence of this syndrome vary greatly. In 1987, the number of people suffering from Usher's syndrome was thought to be only about five in every 100 000. But a much higher incidence than this has been estimated in populations in Finland, Norway and parts of he USA.

Boys and girls can be equally affected. Amongst children in schools for the profoundly deaf, Usher's syndrome is to be found in as many as 10% of these children, so it is an important cause of severe hearing loss.

Some children who have been diagnosed as having Usher's syndrome also show signs of mental instability and/or learning disability. When these added problems are noted the disorder is termed Hallgren's syndrome. The exact connection between these two syndromes is not clear.

CAUSATION

Usher's syndrome is inherited in an autosomally recessive manner. Some children have the added disability of poor balance. This again may be a variant of Usher's syndrome or may have a different basic cause with possible different modes of inheritance.

Recently, abnormalities in the levels of polyunsaturated fatty acids have been found, so Usher's syndrome may yet prove to be a metabolic disorder.

There is no antenatal test available.

CHARACTERISTICS

Usher's syndrome mainly affects two systems of the body – hearing and vision. (The exception to this, of course, is when the other problems associated with Hallgren's syndrome are present.)

Hearing: 90% of babies with Usher's syndrome are born with a profound hearing loss. It is important that this severe problem is detected as soon as possible so that appropriate action can be taken early. In some places routine testing of new-born babys' hearing is practised, which is ideal. Routine tests of hearing later – at around seven to nine months of age – will pick up deafness, but it must be remembered that parents may often suspect that their baby is not hearing properly long before the opportunity for routine testing comes around, so testing should take place earlier if this is the case. Lack of response to loud sudden noises or delay in response to voice should alert all carers of young babies to the possibility of a congenital deafness. The deafness is of a sensori-neural type.

If Usher's syndrome has been diagnosed in a close family member, any suspicion of deafness in a new member must be taken seriously.

Vision is normal at birth in the baby with Usher's syndrome, and also for the first few years of life. But at around ten years of age, the child may discover that he/she is unable to see as well in the dark as his/her contemporaries. Peripheral vision may also begin to become limited. This can be suspected if the child is becoming unaware of objects or people beside him/her when looking straight ahead. This is due to pigmentation of the retina. In Usher's syndrome this takes the form of 'spicule' concretions of abnormal pigment being laid down in the retina. Other pathological changes are also seen in this part of the eye, and these two factors are responsible for a much reduced visual acuity. Vision will become gradually more and more reduced until complete blindness results. This tragedy occurs certainly before the middle years of life, and in many cases earlier than this.

Glaucoma, a dangerously high pressure inside the eyeball, can also occur in Usher's syndrome, and must be remembered when caring for a child with this condition. Here, pain in the eye, rapid blurring of vision and maybe seeing 'haloes' around sources of light are the signs to watch for.

Cataracts can also add to the visual problems of sufferers from Usher's syndrome.

Only about 10% of children with Usher's syndrome will have minimal hearing and visual problems in early childhood. By puberty, however, the hearing loss becomes obvious and gradually worsens, and the pigmentation of the retina makes its appearance, so that vision also declines.

With the relatively high frequency of Usher's syndrome amongst profoundly deaf children, night and peripheral vision should be checked in all severely deaf children.

Ataxia, or poor balance, is sometimes also associated with Usher's syndrome. Children with this manifestation will, for example, find difficulty in turning quickly and in balancing on one foot – movements which their peers can perform easily. This problem does not always occur, but can be an added factor to be remembered when the diagnosis of Usher's syndrome is being queried.

MANAGEMENT IMPLICATIONS

Deafness, if present from birth, will require a full audiometric assessment to quantify the exact amount of hearing loss. Early teaching is vital for the development of any speech, and specialist teachers of the deaf must be involved early.

Vision also requires full assessment early in the child's life to establish a base line for his/her visual acuity at this time. Regular routine checks, particularly on night and peripheral vision, should be done on all profoundly deaf children. Night vision lenses can be helpful in the initial stages of the abnormal pigmentation of the retina. Later, other aids for failing vision will become necessary, and eventually blindness will need specialized care and help.

Cataracts, if present, should be removed to maximize any residual vision.

Glaucoma must also be remembered as a possibility, and treated if found to be present.

Parents will need sensitive and continuing counselling as to the likely outcome of their child's inherited condition. Feelings of guilt must be allayed, and help given to minimize the effects of the child's disturbed vision and hearing as they arise.

Schooling should be geared towards vocational training as a deaf/blind adult. This may seem very hard to take at a time when the child still has some residual vision left, but with the knowledge of the progressive nature of the disorder, it is important that all steps should be taken to reduce the impact of blindness when it does occur.

THE FUTURE

The future can be difficult for the sufferers from Usher's syndrome. Most people will be severely disabled, both visually and auditorally, by the time early adulthood is reached. Specialized training and teaching in the early days can reduce later problems. Full explanation of the probable outcome should be given to parents, and later to the sufferers themselves when it is felt that they are ready to receive this.

Usher's syndrome does not reduce lifespan. Genetic counselling will be necessary when reproductive age is reached.

SELF-HELP GROUP

Usher's Syndrome Services
SENSE
11–13 Clifton Terrace
London N4 3SR
(Tel. 0171 272 7774)

Aims and provisions: information and advice; rehabilitation centres; local support groups.

VATER association

INCIDENCE

An 'association' is a grouping of abnormalities arising together more often than is probable by chance. Many systems or organs of the body can be affected, the name being an acronym of the parts of the body affected.

The VATER association is diagnosed when three of the six possible abnormalities are present: Vertebral abnormality; Anal malformation; Trachea defects; Oesophageal defects; Renal problems and Radial limb defects.

There are several hundred known sufferers from this specific association of abnormalities, which was first described in 1973. It is thought that the VATER association is not always recognized as such. Many babies previously described as having 'multiple abnormalities' could well have had the specific grouping of the VATER association.

Boys and girls are seen to be affected in equal numbers.

This condition is more often seen in the children of diabetic mothers.

CAUSATION

The wide-ranging, and often severe, abnormalities of this association of defects could point to a chromosomal abnormality. But no unusual chromosome pattern has been seen in the VATER association.

Most cases have arisen out of the blue, but a few families are known with more than one affected member. Genetic counselling and family studies are advisable after the birth of a baby with this particular grouping of defects.

There is no antenatal test for this condition, although if there are bony abnormalities in the arms these can be visualized during scanning in the pregnancy.

CHARACTERISTICS

Vertebral abnormalities can take many forms, ranging from the vertebrae being fused together to only half a vertebra being present. These defects are more often found in the lower part of the body in the lumbar region. Occasionally, extra vertebrae are present, for example, six or seven lumbar vertebrae instead of the usual five. This excess of vertebrae can also occur higher up the spine in the thoracic region. Here also, extra ribs can sometimes be seen in association with the extra vertebrae. The effects of these abnormalities depend very much on the site and severity of the defect. Sometimes these unusual features are only noted when X-ray examination is being done for another, quite separate, reason.

Anal atresia: In the severest form there is only a dimpling of the skin where the anus should be situated. The lower bowel can be normally formed but does not extend as far as the exterior. Sometimes the anal canal and anus are present, but are very much narrowed and function only with difficulty.

Tracheal defect: Again, the extent and severity of this abnormality can vary. The most severe problems arise when there is an opening (a fistula) between the oesophagus and the trachea. In conjunction with this the oesophagus itself can be small and under-developed. The baby with this type of defect will have severe respiratory problems at birth. Swallowing will also present major difficulties, once again the extent varying with the severity of the anatomical defect.

Renal abnormalities can also occur, and again vary in severity and type. Kidneys may be situated in unusual positions in the abdomen, and 'horseshoe' kidneys are relatively common. Again, effects will vary according to the actual abnormality. Renal failure is a distinct possibility in the early days with the most severe abnormalities in this system of the body.

Radial limb abnormalities: The radius is one of the bones of the forearm, and in some babies with the VATER association this bone is of a small size or can be absent altogether. This can be detected by antenatal scanning.

Occasionally, **heart defects** are also present in this particular association.

For a definite diagnosis of the VATER association to be made, three of the described abnormalities must be present. It must be emphasized that the degree of abnormality, and hence the severity of the effects, can vary enormously.

MANAGEMENT IMPLICATIONS

Respiratory difficulties will be the most apparent, and in urgent need of special care facilities, immediately after birth. Depending on the degree of abnormality, emergency surgery to correct the anatomical defects may be necessary.

Feeding problems may also occur at a slightly later date if the defect in the trachea is connected to the oesophagus.

The **renal** abnormalities again can present serious problems in the neonatal period depending on the severity of the defects. Renal failure is a distinct possibility in some of the babies who have a severe renal abnormality. This, again, will need special care facilities.

The presence of a narrowed or absent **anus** will also need surgical correction in the early days of life.

If the baby can survive all these potential major surgical procedures, and the defects are not so severe as to be irreparable, the outlook is surprisingly good, but renal failure is a continuing possible threat if the kidney abnormalities are present and severe.

The **vertebral** and other possible **bony** abnormalities may give rise to a few problems of mobility later in life. Again, surgical intervention may be needed for proper function. The absence, or defective size of the radius in the arm can cause problems of rotation movements together with difficulties in carrying anything weighty on this arm.

THE FUTURE

It is difficult to be specific as to the future for a baby born with the VATER association. The range of severity and type of defect is so wide that some individuals will be able to lead near normal lives whilst others may be severely physically disabled.

It is rare for the central nervous system to be affected in any way and intellectual function is only very rarely affected. So from this point of view, career choices will be wide.

Lifespan is again dependent on the type and severity of the abnormalities found.

SELF-HELP GROUP

TOFS (Tracheo-Oesophageal Fistula Society)
St George's Centre
91 Victoria Road
Netherfield
Nottingham NG4 2NN
(Tel. 01602 400694)

Aims and provisions: support by letter and telephone; information and advice; fund-raising.

Vitiligo

ALTERNATIVE NAMES

Primary achromia; idiopathic leukoderma.

INCIDENCE

This skin condition can occur at any time of life, but around 50% of cases occur in children before the teenage years. Two separate studies have suggested that the incidence can be as high as one in every 200 people; the amount of skin involved being very variable. Both sexes are thought to be equally affected.

CAUSATION

The exact cause for this skin condition is not known. Some authorities consider it to be an auto-immune disease. If a number of family members are affected, the risk to a child born to a mother who herself has vitiligo is thought to be 50%.

The basic pathology of vitiligo is an absence of melanocytes (the cells in the skin associated with pigmentation) in the areas of skin affected. The reason for this loss is unknown.

CHARACTERISTICS

A varying amount of skin – anywhere on the body – can be affected by vitiligo. These areas of **skin** are completely white. The amount of skin affected is variable, but in the most severe cases half of the body surface has the typical loss of pigment. In children with a dark complexion this feature stands out in sharp contrast to the normal-coloured skin.

There are no known other characteristics associated with this skin condition. It is important, however, to exclude any other auto-immune conditions – such as can affect the thyroid gland, adrenal glands or stomach, for example – as auto-immune conditions frequently affect more than one part of the body.

MANAGEMENT IMPLICATIONS

It is important to protect the de-pigmented areas of skin against **sunburn**. With no protective melanin in the skin severe burning can result from even limited exposure to sunlight. Sunscreen creams of a high protection factor need to be used for even brief exposure to the sun. It must be remembered also, that sunburn can occur even on a cloudy, but bright day.

Children can be unkind to classmates with vitiligo – various names such as 'piebald' being commonly, and unkindly, used. Some sensitive children will respond to this form of **teasing** with a variety of behaviour patterns ranging from school phobia to aggression.

It is important that teachers are aware of the **non-infectious** nature of pupils with vitligo. (Vitiligo can be confused at times with pityriasis alba – a skin condition, probably viral, in which there are temporary de-pigmented areas of skin. This condition will clear within a few weeks with no treatment, whereas vitiligo is a long lasting condition.)

For small areas of de-pigmented skin, **cosmetic creams** can be used, but this is impracticable for larger areas of affected skin.

THE FUTURE

Most cases of vitiligo are life-long, although very occasionally spontaneous remission can occur.

It is important to remember that the de-pigmented areas of skin are more prone to skin cancers, especially in climates that have long days of hot sunshine.

SELF-HELP GROUP

The Vitiligo Society
97 Avenue Road
Beckenham
Kent BR3 4RX
(Tel. 0181 776 7022)

Aims and provisions: mutual support and practical advice for sufferers; fund-raising for research; leaflets and training courses; newsletter. The society has over 1800 members in the UK.

Waardenburg's syndrome

INCIDENCE

This syndrome has three distinct sub-types, depending on the presence and severity of specific characteristics. For example, type 3 has abnormalities of the limbs in addition to the features shown by the other two types. The general overall incidence of the condition, taking all the sub-types into account, is one in every 20 000 to 40 000 births.

The importance of this syndrome lies in the fact that amongst children who are deaf from birth, three in every 100 have Waardenburg's syndrome.

CAUSATION

Waardenburg's syndrome is inherited as an autosomal dominant condition. In a few families having a specific variant of the condition, the inheritance pattern is thought to be a recessive one. There is also some link with a particular form of albinism in this variant.

Boys and girls can be equally affected. It is probable that the affected gene is located on chromosome 9. There is no antenatal test available to determine Waardenburg's syndrome.

CHARACTERISTICS

All the characteristics of Waardenburg's syndrome – apart from type 3 – are confined to the head and neck region.

Almost all children with Waardenburg's syndrome have a specific unusual finding in the shape of their eyes. The inner edge of the eye, instead of being tight up against the bridge of the nose, is displaced outwards. Included in this positioning are the openings of the lower tear-ducts, which are also placed further away from the mid-line of the face than is usual. Whilst this leads to few problems, tears tend to flow less easily than normal.

Eyes can have other very specific striking characteristics. In some children with Waardenburg's syndrome, one eye can be light blue in colour, whist the other eye can be dark brown, if this is the family characteristic eye colour. This can give a most unusual aspect to the appearance of the face. Occasionally, only a small segment of the iris is of a lighter colour, but is still a noticeable characteristic. This feature has no effect on vision.

The only possible visual difficulty seen in Waardenburg's syndrome can be the onset of **glaucoma**, a dangerous increase in tension inside the eyeball. This is probably due to the unusual structure of the orbit, making normal drainage of fluid from the eye difficult.

The **noses** of children with Waardenburg's syndrome are small at birth and tend to remain so throughout life. This can lead to young children in particular having a frequently blocked nose, with more frequent upper respiratory tract infections than usual being the norm. These children are often 'mouth-breathers'.

Along with the unusual eye shape and tiny nose goes an unusual **eyebrow** feature. Eyebrows tend to grow across the forehead until they meet in the middle over the bridge of the nose. Of course, not everyone with confluent eyebrows has Waardenburg's syndrome, but this feature is yet one more sign that can confirm a diagnosis of the syndrome.

Hair: one of the most striking features of Waardenburg's syndrome (especially when occurring in conjunction with different coloured eyes) is a completely white 'forelock'. This can be present at birth, even in a baby with a dark head of hair. Occasionally, this unusual colouring disappears during early childhood, only to reappear again during the teenage years. Early greying of all facial hair, eyebrows and eyelashes as well as hair on the head, has also been reported, not just in the twenties but as early as seven years of age!

Deafness is the most serious of the features of Waardenburg's syndrome. This characteristic affects up to one-quarter of all sufferers from the condition. The deafness is present from birth, and can affect both ears or only one. It is a sensori-neural type, in which the actual nerves of hearing are affected. It is vitally important that the deafness is recognized early so that speech, and many other aspects of normal development, are not secondarily affected. Regrettably, in the past, some profoundly deaf children have been 'labelled' as having learning disability – and treated as such. With today's knowledge of normal child development and screening procedures this should not occur.

These are the usual signs of all the types of Waardenburg's syndrome. Children with type 3 may have developmental abnormalities of their upper limbs, in addition. This may take the form of a generalized lack of antenatal growth of the arms. Alternatively, there may be abnormalities of the fingers; either extra fingers being present or two or more fingers being fused together. Here, of course, there will be problems of fine, precise movement.

MANAGEMENT IMPLICATIONS

It is important that Waardenburg's syndrome is recognized early in a child's life so that hearing and vision can be checked.

Routine checks on **hearing** from an early age should pick up any hearing loss. Serious note should always be taken when parents suggest that their baby is not hearing properly. Very special care must be taken, under these circumstances, to check hearing thoroughly and to continue to do so, at regular intervals. If the baby is shown to be profoundly deaf, referral to a service for hearing impaired children (if available) is important. Early help is vital if speech is to be attained at all. Later in childhood, special educational facilities for deaf children may be needed if the deafness is bilateral and profound. Lesser degrees of hearing loss may also need speech therapy input, and also complete hearing assessment.

Vision: the important condition to be aware of is glaucoma. Pain in the child's eye, blurred vision or reports of 'haloes' around lights are all pointers to the need for urgent visual assessment. Eyedrops or surgery may be necessary if the pressure in the eye is found to be raised.

THE FUTURE

This will largely depend on the presence or otherwise, of hearing problems. If this is not present, all the other features of eye colour, white forelock and unusual eye-shape will all point to a lesser manifestation of the syndrome. These latter characteristics will have no bearing on either career choice or leisure activities – in fact they can be added attractive features!

Sometimes the more minor aspects of Waardenburg's syndrome are only recognized after a more severely affected family member has been investigated.

SELF-HELP GROUP

There is no specific group for Waardenburg's syndrome, but if deafness is a marked feature the following can be of help:

National Deaf Childrens Society
45 Hereford Road
London W2 5AH
(Tel. 0171 250 0123)

West's syndrome

ALTERNATIVE NAMES

Infantile spasms; hypsarrhythmia.

INCIDENCE

The exact incidence of West's syndrome is difficult to determine, as it merges with other types of epilepsy, of which there are many. It is only when specific tests are carried out, and the results added to the typical clinical signs, that this syndrome can be distinguished.

CAUSATION

This syndrome is due to the baby's immature brain reacting to any one of a number of factors. These can range from lack of oxygen at birth to infections in the early days of life, such as meningitis or some injury to the brain. In a significant number of babies with West's syndrome some developmental abnormality in the brain is also found.

Other possibilities as to the cause of this particular syndrome can be some disturbance of metabolism which in turn has an effect on the young brain. Examples of this are phenylketonuria, in which there is abnormal metabolism of the amino acid, phenyl-alanine; hypoglycaemia, in which there is a low blood sugar for some reason, or low levels of pyridoxine (a vitamin of the B group).

The common factor in all these possible causes is that the result is a failure of development of the normal organization of the electrical activity of the brain. This results in the typical convulsions seen in West's syndrome.

Obviously, in many cases there is no direct inheritance pattern involved if the cause is thought to be an outside event, such as infection or lack of oxygen at a critical time, but if the cause is found to be metabolic, the most usual pattern of inheritance is autosomal recessive.

CHARACTERISTICS

Babies with West's syndrome usually have no problems at birth. However, if the birth has been difficult, and lack of oxygen is a marked feature, this may be one of the precipitating causes for the condition. (Some authorities describe two distinct types, one occurring before six months of age (about 10%), and the other type after this age. The latter is thought to be due possibly to an unrecognized encephalitis or to an underlying defect in the metabolism in the brain. In the latter type the child subsequently has good motor skills, but often has difficulties with language.)

Fits of a particular nature will begin to occur at any time between the early neonatal days and two years of life. The most usual time of onset is between three and eight months of life. The fits are of a specific type. The baby will jerk into a flexed position and then rapidly return to the normal way of lying. These fits can occur in rapid succession. Sometimes it is only the baby's head that is involved, a nodding motion being the only indication that a fit is occurring. This type of fit is also known as hypsarrythmia, and can be seen as such on an EEG tracing. Sixty per cent of babies with West's syndrome show this typical tracing when an EEG is recorded.

Before the onset of the fits the baby may be developing normally, showing all the usual normal developmental steps of smiling, head control etc. in a normal sequence. Other babies with the syndrome may already be exhibiting some developmental delay.

One fairly frequent feature which is noticed to precede a fit is a decrease in the baby's visual alertness. He/she will not respond as readily to visual stimuli as do babies of a similar age or, indeed, as quickly as he/she had done previously.

The spasms, or fits, commonly occur shortly after the baby awakes from sleep, and a rapid succession of fits may follow this first fit. CAT scans have shown 60% of babies with West's syndrome to have some abnormality of the brain. This can range from a generalized atrophy of this organ to specific abnormalities in certain parts of the brain (cf Aicardi's syndrome).

It is important to exclude a metabolic cause for this syndrome. Specific tests for metabolic disease should, therefore, be done – tests for abnormalities in the metabolism of certain amino acids and also pyridoxine, for example.

Treatment to control the frequent spasms is with ACTH. This can effectively control the fits, but relapse can occur, giving rise to the need for a further course of ACTH.

The outlook for babies with West's syndrome is variable. Ten percent of babies initially suffering this type of fit will develop normally, and have no permanent after-effects. The remainder will be left with varying degrees of learning disability, and 50% of these children will go on to develop other types of seizures as they get older.

There are no other developmental abnormalities to be seen with West's syndrome.

MANAGEMENT IMPLICATIONS

It is important that West's syndrome is diagnosed as early as possible, so that a course of treatment can begin. The fits are quite specific clinically, and the EEG tracing will confirm this.

Developmental checks should be performed routinely, preferably by a multidisciplinary team, throughout the early childhood years. Specific areas of delay can then be helped by physiotherapy and speech therapy, for example. Specialized teaching in the pre-school years is also valuable in helping the child learn self-help skills.

Schooling will need to be geared to the abilities of each individual child as recorded after developmental testing.

The subsequent development of other types of fits unfortunately seen in about 50% of children with West's syndrome will need assessment to determine the best anti-convulsant drug, or combination of drugs, necessary to control the fits.

Parents will need sensitive counselling, and information as to the probable cause behind their child's illness. Respite care facilities, if available, are also important. In this way, parents and any other children in the family can have a holiday together without the continual worry of a disabled family member.

THE FUTURE

Ten percent of children with West's syndrome as babies will be able to lead normal lives with no sequelae following on from their difficult first days of life. Genetic counselling is advisable once reproductive age is reached. Regrettably, the remainder of children with this syndrome will have varying degrees of learning disability for the rest of their lives. This will, of course, influence any choice of career, and the most severely disabled will need full-time care for the rest of their lives.

Life expectancy is within the normal range.

SELF-HELP GROUP

West's Syndrome Support Group
8 Waddon Close
Croydon
Surrey CR0 4JT
(Tel. 0181 680 8449)

Aims and provisions: links with other affected families.

William's syndrome

ALTERNATIVE NAME

Infantile hypercalcaemia.

INCIDENCE

The estimated number of babies suffering from this syndrome has only recently been reported, and is thought to be in the region of one in every 10 000 born. Boys and girls can be affected equally.

CAUSATION

William's syndrome was thought to arise only as a sporadic new mutation, but recently it has been suggested that the condition may be inherited as an autosomal dominant.

The basic pathology is one of a fault in calcium metabolism, which leads to an excess of calcium in the body as a whole. If not corrected, this can affect brain cells and lead to a degree of learning disability.

CHARACTERISTICS

Facial features are quite typical for all William's syndrome sufferers. Children with this syndrome will have round, chubby faces with full lips and a tip-tilted nose.

During infancy, babies with William's syndrome often **fail to grow** at the normal rate. Their birth weight is often on the low side, and they are seen to grow slowly, usually along, or below, the third centile line on the standard growth charts. Excessive vomiting can also be a feature, adding to the problems of adequate weight gain.

Sleeping can also be a problem. Parents can become completely worn out by their restless, demanding baby who, in addition to not gaining weight along the usual lines, does not seem to want to sleep, either. This sleeplessness continues into later childhood.

Along with this lack of the normal sleep pattern, goes a good deal of **hyperactivity** during the day, adding to the parents' difficulties of getting adequate rest.

Behavioural problems are also commonly seen, and as the William's syndrome child gets older he/she becomes increasingly verbally able. This adds to the parents' problems, as the child appears to be older and more able than is really the case. All in all, children with William's syndrome can be extraordinarily difficult to handle.

Heart defects also frequently occur, the most often seen abnormality being aortic stenosis – a narrowing of the large blood vessel leaving the heart. Other structural defects in the cardiovascular system are also seen more often than is usual.

Hearing: It has been reported that children with William's syndrome seem to be especially susceptible to loud noise, and find any excess of noise very distressing.

A further complication of the high calcium levels found in this condition may be that the child may suffer, at a comparatively early age, from **renal calculi**, or kidney 'stones' – those accretions of calcium which can be so excruciatingly painful as they pass down the ureter into the bladder.

MANAGEMENT IMPLICATIONS

The **failure to thrive** in infancy will need patience to ensure that the baby obtains adequate nutrition in spite of the persistent vomiting and general hyperactive behaviour. Dietetic advice is essential to know which are the most suitable foods to offer the baby with William's syndrome. For example, foods low in vitamin D and calcium are advisable if the high levels of calcium in the blood persist. This early difficult feeding stage usually improves with maturity, although episodes of hypercalcaemia can recur in later life. Nevertheless, many children with William's syndrome do not achieve a normal adult height, but are always on the short side of normal.

Heart defects, if severe and causing symptoms, may need cardiac surgery. The on-going care of a cardiologist is always advisable.

Education will very much depend on the child's abilities, as well as how well the behavioural problems are under control. Individual educational programmes, best suited to each child's range of ability, are the ideal.

Activities which use up some of the abundant energy seen in the child with William's syndrome are a 'must'. Shorter periods of teaching than normal will accommodate the child's short attention span and also allow time for his/her verbal loquacity! Also, it must not be forgotten that it is all too easy to think of the child with William's syndrome as more able than he/she really is, due to the extreme ease with which he/she uses words and language. It is only when practical concepts need to be put into practice that the child will find difficulty.

THE FUTURE

Career choices must be carefully evaluated for the school-leaver with William's syndrome. His/her undoubted verbal abilities must not be allowed to hide the true nature of the young person's problems as he/she attempts to cope with the stresses of the adult world.

Life expectancy can be limited by cardiac defects or by the side effects from the high calcium levels in the body, such as the renal problems.

SELF-HELP GROUPS

Infantile Hypercalcaemia Foundation Ltd
Mulberry Cottage
37 Mulberry Green
Old Harlow
Essex CM17 0EY
(Tel. 01279 427214)

Aims and provisions: parent support, information and advice on the syndrome; national and regional meetings; guidelines and newsletter for parents and teachers.

Advice and help can also be given by:

Research Trust for Metabolic Disease in Childhood (RTMDC)
Golden Gates Lodge
Weston Road
Crewe
Cheshire CW1 1XN
(Tel. 01272 250221)

Wolf–Hirschhorn syndrome

ALTERNATIVE NAMES

Wolf syndrome; partial chromosome 4 deletion syndrome.

INCIDENCE

This is a very rare syndrome, but around 120 cases have been confirmed in the literature. Of these cases, two-thirds have been girls, although babies of either sex can be affected. A number of still-born babies have also been found to be affected by this chromosomal defect.

HISTORY

Both Wolf and Hirschhorn described this syndrome in 1965.

CAUSATION

The Wolf–Hirschhorn syndrome results from the loss of some of the genetic material on the short arm of chromosome 4. In most cases this abnormality arises spontaneously, but in around 10% of cases the syndrome arises as the result of a 'balanced translocation'. It is important that the parent's chromosomes are examined for the presence of this translocation as future pregnancies may also be affected.

The age of either parent seems to have no effect on the occurrence of this syndrome.

Chorionic villus sampling can detect this condition in the baby if performed between the ninth and 12th weeks of pregnancy.

CHARACTERISTICS

The baby with the Wolf–Hirschhorn syndrome will have a **low birth weight**, even though the pregnancy has continued to the full 40 weeks. This lack of adequate growth continues after birth, weightgain being very slow in spite of adequate feeding.

The **facial features** of the baby are quite distinctive, including:

- a small head – **microcephaly**;
- there is no usual indentation of the **nose** between the eyebrows, there being a continuous line from the forehead to the tip of the nose. This feature has been graphically described as resembling a Greek helmet, the flat bridge of the baby's nose closely akin to the protective nose-piece of this ancient piece of armour;
- the **eyes** are widely spaced, and there may also be a squint present;
- the **upper lip** is short;
- the **ears** are low-set.

The baby with the Wolf–Hirschhorn syndrome will be **floppy** at birth, and the muscle tone will always be weak. 'Milestones' of motor movement will usually be delayed.

Seizures are a frequent occurrence and can be difficult to control.

Learning disability is usually severe.

Other characteristics can also be present, although they do not necessarily occur in every baby with this syndrome:

- **Heart defects**, of different types, can occur;
- A **cleft palate** and/or **lip** can be an immediately obvious feature;
- The **testes** can be small and undescended, and a **hypospadias** can be present.

MANAGEMENT IMPLICATIONS

Feeding difficulties and **lack of weight gain** can be worrying problems during the early days of life. This is due both to the poor muscle tone as well as a continuation of the inadequate growth seen in the antenatal days. Also, if a cleft palate and/or lip is present the feeding difficulties are magnified by these anatomical features. Small, frequent feeds will be necessary initially, with early referral to a dental department for the best method of treatment of the specific cleft palate. Nasogastric feeding may be necessary for some severely affected babies.

Any **heart defect** will need to diagnosed and assessed, together with appropriate treatment should heart failure occur at any time during the early days of life, due to a severe heart problem.

Surgical treatment for the **cleft palate and/or lip**, if they are present will be necessary. The timing of these operative procedures will depend on the physical state of the baby due to other problems.

Seizures will need to be controlled with anti-convulsant drugs. In many cases, finding the right drug, or combination of drugs, can prove difficult. Several drugs may need to be tried before the most helpful one is found.

Regular **developmental checks** must be carried out to determine the level of learning disability as well as the development of motor skills. When school-age is reached, the appropriate schooling for each individual child needs to be considered with the help both of health and education authorities.

At a later date the **hypospadias**, if present, will need to be corrected surgically if problems are encountered by the boy being unable to direct the flow of urine.

Parents will need **support** both during the early stages of their baby's life and as they come to terms with his/her disability. Later, **respite care** will be necessary, particularly if there are other children in the family to consider. A week or two away from the demanding needs of a severely disabled family member can do much for the morale and physical well-being of the whole family

Genetic counselling is important if the parents are considering further pregnancies. If a balanced translocation is found, investigations at an early stage in future pregnancies will be needed.

THE FUTURE

Many babies with the most profound defects do not survive the first year of life, but if they do, a life of severe disability will be the regretful outlook. The average lifespan is not known, but certainly the teenage years can be attained, and adults with this syndrome have been reported.

An independent lifestyle can, unfortunately, never be attained.

SELF-HELP GROUP

Wolf–Hirschhorn Support Group
26 Harvester's Close
Rainham
Kent ME8 8PA
(Tel. 01634 372218)

Aims and provisions: information about the condition; contact between parents of children with the Wolf-Hirschhorn syndrome; liaison between professionals and researchers into the syndrome.

Appendix A: Background genetics

Knowledge of genetics has increased by leaps and bounds from the time when Gregor Mendel – an Austrian monk and botanist – laid the foundation for the science with his experiments on peas in the mid-19th century. His work lay dormant for many years, but was eventually revived and found to be a correct assessment of the basis of some types of inheritance. Crick and Watson, in Cambridge in the 1950s, further advanced knowledge with their description of the way in which DNA was arranged in a double helix to carry the chemical building bricks of life. Following on from these discoveries, genetics has become an ever-increasingly precise science.

Genes and chromosomes are the 'life-blood' of the geneticist! But just what are these tiny pieces of matter that have such overwhelming effects, for good or ill, on human life?

Genes, of which there are up to 100 000 in each human being, consist of chemicals, known as 'bases'. These are arranged in a strict order on the chromosomes and are read off in a three-base code containing the instructions to make proteins. Diseases can be caused by alterations (mutations) in the genetic code itself, either by the order of the bases being changed or by the code being altered in some way; a part being deleted, for example. (Chromosomes can be seen through a microscope, but genes are too tiny to be visualized.)

Chromosomes (meaning, literally, a 'coloured body', due to the fact that they are able to take up certain coloured stains) are to be found in every cell in the human body – of which there are billions. The nucleus of each cell houses these distinctive thread-like structures. Each cell in the body normally has 46 chromosomes (22 pairs known as 'autosomes' and one pair of sex chromosomes) with the exception of the sex cells – the ovum and the sperm. These latter cells, having the important function of reproduction, only have 23 chromosomes each. (These sex chromosomes are denoted X and Y; males have one X and one Y chromosome (XY), whilst females have two X chromosomes (XX).) At fertilization, these sex cells combine to make a new individual, who thus receives the full complement of 46 chromosomes.

The process by which the sex cells obtain their lessened complement of chromosomes is in the way the cells divide to produce the sperm and ovum – or 'gametes' – containing their diminished complement of only 23 chromosomes. This process is known as **meiosis**, and fulfils the task of 'shuffling' the genes, so that a widely varying set of characteristics are dealt out to each child, making that child completely different from any other individual. (Some forms of twins are a special case.)

This method of cell division is quite different from the way in which other body cells divide to produce more cells for growth and repair. This latter process is known as **mitosis**, and here each daughter cell produced is an exact copy of the parent cell, each with 46 chromosomes.

It is during the process of meiosis that chromosomes can become damaged or the sequencing of genes can become upset. These variations, depending on just what they are, and where they occur, will set the scene for the specific characteristics for each new individual produced at conception.

The individual pairs of chromosomes are defined by way of their size, shape and other characteristics and the pairs are numbered from one to 23 for ease of referral.

The majority of syndromes have a genetic basis, and there are three main ways in which this can happen.

- There may be a **single gene** at fault, where the bases making up the gene have been disordered or mutated.
- There may be **chromosomal abnormalities**, involving whole chromosomes or segments, or segments may be moved, that is 'translocated', onto a different chromosome.
- A **genetic predisposition** may be inherited which, together with other environmental factors, will result in a particular characteristic or disease pattern.

SINGLE GENE DISORDERS

At each position, or locus, on each chromosome is a pair of genes specific to a certain characteristic, for example, blue or brown eyes, curly or straight hair as well as more wide-ranging, and perhaps, serious disorders. If one of the pair becomes altered (by a mistake in the sequence, for example a 'mutation') this may give rise to specific syndromes, with specific recognizable characteristics. When the gene causing a disease is on one of the autosomal chromosomes the condition is said to be **autosomally** inherited. In practice this means that any abnormal gene on a particular chromosome can affect males and females equally.

Alternatively, when the gene is on one of the sex chromosomes, the condition is said to be **sex-linked**. For all practical purposes all sex-linked inherited conditions are **X-linked**, that is, carried on the X chromosome. This means that the **carrier** of a specific condition will always be a female, and each son has an equal chance of inheriting her normal or abnormal gene. This process of inheritance will also mean that each daughter will also have an equal chance of being a carrier of the genetically determined characteristic.

Autosomally inherited characteristics can be passed to the next generation in two different ways; either as a **dominant** characteristic, or as a **recessive characteristic**.

In a dominant mode of inheritance one of the parents themselves will show the features of the disease or characteristic. There is a 50% chance that, under these circumstances, each pregnancy will result in an affected child. (It is a common fallacy that if two parents with the specific genetic make-up for a particular disease had two children with the characteristics of the disorder, any succeeding children would not have the condition. The 50% chance has already been fulfilled. This is, regrettably, not the case, as the chances are 50% for **each** pregnancy.)

In a recessive disorder, neither parent will be affected with the characteristics of the syndrome or disease. But if two people who are each carrying the recessive gene have children, there is a 25% chance that an affected child will result from the union. As with the dominant mode of inheritance, each succeeding pregnancy will run the risk of an affected child.

A few examples of these Mendelian forms of inheritance will help to make the inheritance patterns clear.

Autosomal dominant conditions (e.g. neurofibromatosis)

An example of a family tree, through three generations, is shown in Figure A.1. Both males and females are affected in this mode of inheritance. Breaking the picture down to what is actually happening in the cells will show the way in which autosomal dominant characteristics are brought about (Figure A.2).

In these circumstances any individual with A will show the characteristics of the condition. The 50% chance of inheritance can be seen.

There are a number of factors, however, which can influence this seemingly straightforward inheritance picture.

The severity of the condition, which has been dominantly inherited, can vary widely within members of the same family – some showing fewer characteristics than others.

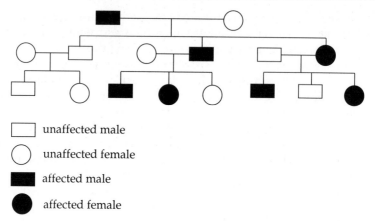

unaffected male

unaffected female

affected male

affected female

Figure A.1 Typical family tree of an autosomal dominant condition.

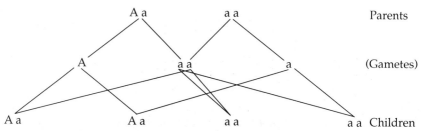

Figure A.2 Genetic make-up of an autosomal dominant condition; 'A' = the altered gene of the dominant condition, 'a' = the normal gene.

Unfortunately, a mildly affected parent will not always have a child who is similarly mildly affected. He or she may manifest the disorder in a very severe form. Examples of this variable **expressivity** can be seen in two conditions – tuberous sclerosis and neurofibromatosis. In the former condition, a mildly affected parent may have only the typical rash of the syndrome on his/her face. But he/she could have a child severely affected with all the other characteristics of the syndrome. Similarly, a parent with only minimal signs of neurofibromatosis, such as an excess of freckles in the armpit, could have a child with many of the more serious manifestations of the disorder.

The parent, or indeed anyone in the family, may not suffer from the condition at all. But a child can be born, to unaffected parents, with a specific syndrome due to a new **mutation**. In this circumstance there is a change in the structure of a particular gene. Neurofibromatosis, for example, can also arise in this manner as well as being inherited. Achondroplasia is a further disorder that commonly occurs as a new mutation. The age of the parents has some bearing on this aspect of dominant inheritance. Under these circumstances the parents of the affected child are not usually at any increased risk of giving birth to a further child with the same condition, but the child himself/herself will stand the usual 50% chance of having affected children.

Some diseases, such as Huntington's chorea, do not manifest themselves until middle life, so children can be born before the parents are aware that such a condition is part of their genetic make-up.

Autosomal recessive conditions (e.g. cystic fibrosis)

An example of a typical family tree, through three generations, for an autosomal recessive disorder, is shown in Figure A.3.

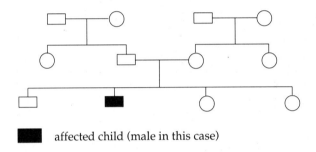

■ affected child (male in this case)

Figure A.3 Typical family tree of an autosomal recessive condition.

Here there are no clues from the pedigree, as the disease was only known to be inherited once the diagnosis was made. But the pedigree can be interpreted as in Figure A.4 to show who is a carrier.

Again, both males and females can be affected by this mode of inheritance. There is a 25% chance of a child being born with the condition. Two of four children will be carriers, whilst one in four will be unaffected. Again, breaking the picture down further, as in Figure A.5, will show how this is brought about.

In these circumstances, an individual with bb as their genetic make-up will have the condition, whilst those people with Bb will be carriers, and those with BB will be unaffected.

The commonest condition with an autosomal recessive inheritance in Caucasian races is cystic fibrosis – the disease being virtually unknown in other parts of the world. About one person in 20 within this population is a carrier for this disorder. Other conditions which have an autosomal recessive disorder are, for example, Friedrich's ataxia, Hurler's syndrome, and phenylketonuria.

Autosomal recessive disorders occur more frequently where there is **consanguinity** (close blood relationship) between the parents – as in first-cousin marriages, for example. The reason for this is that the parents

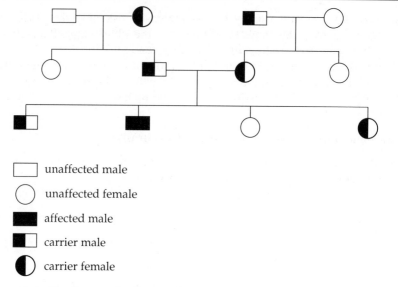

☐ unaffected male

○ unaffected female

■ affected male

◧ carrier male

◑ carrier female

Figure A.4 Family tree showing carrier status.

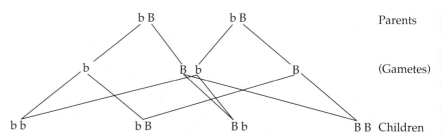

Figure A.5 Genetic make-up of an autosomal recessive condition; 'b' = the altered gene of the recessive condition, 'B' = the normal gene.

more likely to have a similar genetic make-up due to their common ancestors.

X-linked recessive conditions (e.g. haemophilia)

In this form of inheritance, the X chromosome carries the altered gene. Males are affected, with the condition being transmitted through a healthy female carrier. An example of a typical family tree is shown in Figure A.6.

This kind of pedigree would raise suggestions that an X-linked disorder is involved and this proves to be the case. The pedigree can be interpreted as in Figure A.7 to show who is a carrier.

Breaking the picture down into the gametes will make this initial complicated picture clearer (Figure A.8).

There is a (50%) chance that a boy will be affected.

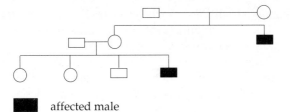

Figure A.6 Typical family tree of an X-linked recessive condition.

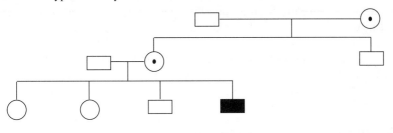

Figure A.7 Family tree showing carrier status.

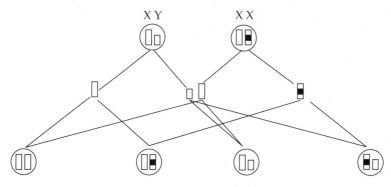

Fig A.8

Figure A.8 Genetic make-up of an X-linked recessive condition.

There are many conditions which have an X-linked recessive type of inheritance, such as haemophilia (probably the most well-known), Hunter's syndrome and Duchenne muscular dystrophy.

Daughters of men who have an X-linked recessive condition will of necessity be carriers of the condition, but none of his sons will be affected.

At present, there have been no Y-linked syndromes described.

There are nearly 4000 traits (fortunately not all producing symptoms of disease!) that are thought to be controlled by single genes. Over 2000 of these have already been mapped to specific places on the chromosomes, and more are being added weekly. Gene-mapping is an important part of antenatal diagnosis, carrier detection and potential treatment of genetic disease. Single gene disorders account for around 1 % of all congenital anomalies.

CHROMOSOMAL ABNORMALITIES

As each chromosome carries a huge number of genes, an abnormality in a small part of the chromosome can have far-reaching effects in many parts of the body, involving many systems.

There are two main groups into which chromosomal abnormalities can be divided: **numerical**, in which there are too many, or too few, chromosomes present in the individual with the syndrome; and **structural**, where, for example, part of the chromosome can be missing or altered.

Numerical abnormalities

These generally arise if chromosomes pair together during meiosis (when ova and sperm are made). At this time, one of the chromosomes fails to separate at a critical stage of meiosis. In Down's syndrome this involves chromosome 21 with the result that there are three chromosomes present.

Two further examples of numerical chromosomal abnormalities are Edward's syndrome, in which there are three number 18 chromosomes, and Patau syndrome in which there are three number 13 chromosomes. Children with both these conditions are very severely physically disabled and have severe learning disability.

Turner's syndrome has a different numerical abnormality. This syndrome, which only affects girls, has one too few chromosomes, one of the X chromosomes being absent. The sex chromosomes can also show other numerical abnormalities. For example, Klinefelter's syndrome sufferers have an extra X chromosome, making their genetic make-up XXY, leading to specific characteristics.

Structural abnormalities

These can involve any chromosome, one of the commonest faults being a **deletion** of part of a chromosome. An example of this is in some cases of Prader–Willi syndrome in which a small part of the long arm of chromosome 15 is missing.

The fragile X syndrome is so named because it has been noted to have a particular appearance at the end of the long arm of the X chromosome – it looks as if the end is about to become detached because of a structural change.

These abnormalities can give rise to far-reaching effects on the person with this kind of genetic make-up.

Translocation, or movement of one piece of a specific chromosome onto a different chromosome, also gives rise to very specific characteristics in each case.

A **balanced translocation** occurs when pieces from two chromosomes break and exchange places, leaving the same amount of genetic material present. This will have no effect on the individual but can lead to profound effects on their children.

Chromosomal abnormalities are found in 0.6% of live born children. Not perhaps a great number at first sight, but nevertheless much heartache and disability results from these tiny differences in genetic make-up. Many chromosomal disorders, particularly the numerical ones, such as Down's syndrome, have a higher incidence when mothers are older.

Antenatal diagnosis of chromosomal abnormalities is possible at around ten weeks of pregnancy using the technique of chorionic villus sampling, which is described in the final section.

GENETIC PREDISPOSITION (OR MULTI-FACTORIAL INHERITANCE)

This is the largest group of genetic factors causing abnormality. Here there is a familial tendency to a particular condition, but this does not follow the usual laws of Mendelian inheritance as is seen in the single gene causes of abnormality. Other factors, such as environmental ones, both antenatally and postnatally, can have a bearing on whether the disease manifests itself openly or not. There can also be more than one genetic factor at work under these conditions, i.e. unlike the single gene fault, several genes can be altered in a less serious way. Probably everyone can think of some condition which is more common in their particular family than in their neighbour's family. This can be as trivial as a particular way of walking or as serious as a tendency to a specific cancer. Such a relatively common condition as coronary heart disease would appear to have a genetic component which, when added to 'environmental' factors, such as being over-weight, smoking etc. leads to acute disease. Diabetes and schizophrenia show a similar genetic predisposition. Much research is being carried out to determine the genetic content of these disorders.

These, briefly, are the genetic ways in which certain specific syndromes can arise, but there is one further way in which abnormalities – giving rise to specific syndromes – can occur. These are the events which can occur during pregnancy, damaging development of the baby, and can lead to profound life-long problems. There are a number of examples of this, and probably two of the most well-known are the 'rubella syndrome' baby and the 'foetal alcohol syndrome' baby. Here, although the genetic inheritance of the baby may have been perfect, he/she can be born with a clutch of recognizable specific symptoms and signs. These are due, in the first case, to an attack of rubella (German measles) in the mother during the early days of her pregnancy, and in the latter case, excess alcohol intake during pregnancy. Drugs other than alcohol, can also have a variety of deleterious effects on the foetus if taken during a critical stage of development. The thalidamide tragedy is one example.

Coming into the world is no easy matter. When one takes into account the pitfalls of genetic inheritance, environmental factors both antenatally and after birth, together with all the potentially fatal infections that abound, it is a miracle that anyone lives for one hour – let alone three score years and ten, or more!

Nowadays genetic disease can be predicted to a far greater extent than was possible even a decade ago. With greater understanding of inheritance patterns, screening during pregnancy for families at risk of genetically determined conditions can detect problems at an early stage in the unborn baby. If a severe disability is diagnosed by these methods, the parents can consider a number of choices including whether to end the pregnancy.

If a child with a genetic condition has already been born to a family, **genetic counselling**, before a further pregnancy is embarked upon, can give parents an idea as to the possibility of a further child being born with the same condition. This counselling (by a doctor especially interested, and trained, in genetics) will involve taking a detailed family history – possibly going back several generations. Such information can prove highly useful. For example, a family with a boy who has been diagnosed as having Duchenne muscular dystrophy may be able to remember, when questioned specifically, an uncle who died at a young age, and who was in a wheelchair for the latter part of his life. The chances are that this uncle, too, was a Duchenne muscular dystrophy sufferer. So, the pedigree confirms the mode of inheritance. The family thus informed will be in a better position to decide either not to have any further children or to accept the risk of a possibly affected child being born. If the latter course is decided upon, various methods of screening for abnormalities during pregnancy can be used if they wish.

SCREENING TESTS DURING PREGNANCY

Blood tests

These tests on the mother-to-be's blood have a limited use, but can give certain valuable information in specific instances. With spina bifida babies, and other similar conditions where there are potential problems in the development of the baby's nervous system, the levels of alpha-fetoprotein in the mother's blood will be higher than normal. These high levels are not in themselves sufficiently reliable to be quite certain of the diagnosis, as they can be high in certain other disorders, but the need for further investigation by ultra-sonic screening and/or amniocentesis will be shown.

Alpha-fetoprotein levels in the mother's blood can also be a valuable indicator that a Down's syndrome baby may have been conceived. Levels under these circumstances are low. The triple test, in which three factors are estimated (oestriol and chorionic gonadotrophin levels as well as that of alpha-fetoprotein) can give useful pointers.

Ultra-sound scanning

This technique uses ultra-sonic waves (sound waves too high be heard by the human ear) which are reflected by the unborn baby's body to form patterns which can be visualized on a 'television' screen. Skeletal abnormalities can be seen and compared against known normal values for the age of the unborn baby. For example, the abnormal limbs of a baby with Cornelia de Lange syndrome may be diagnosed in this way.

The continuing normal growth of a baby can also be estimated by serial scans, paying particular attention to head growth. Possible anatomical heart defects can also be visualized by this method. Ultra-sound is widely used in obstetric departments, and is a safe, useful tool in prenatal diagnosis.

Amniocentesis

A sample of the amniotic fluid surrounding the baby in the bag of membranes in the uterus can be taken and analysed. This is done under local anaesthesia through the mother's abdominal wall. Analysis of the withdrawn fluid and/or cells can identify a number of chromosomal defects and metabolic diseases in the baby. Amniocentesis is usually done at 16 weeks of pregnancy but in some centres may be performed at about 13 weeks.

Chorionic villus sampling

This is a comparatively new technique performed at between nine and 12 weeks of pregnancy which can be used to identify single gene, chromosomal and metabolic disorders in the unborn baby. The actual cells removed during this test are cells from the placenta. These cells are made from the developing embryo soon after fertilization has taken place and so are of the same origin as the baby's own body cells, and therefore, representative of his/her genetic make-up. This procedure is done earlier in pregnancy than amniocentesis. Decisions can thus be taken earlier regarding possible termination of the pregnancy if a severe abnormality has been found.

Genetics is a young, fascinating science – albeit a complex one. The basis for many inherited conditions, as well as the potential for future disease, is rapidly becoming known. Ethical dangers obviously abound with this increase in knowledge, but it is to be hoped that the result of genetic investigation will only be good.

Appendix B: Regional genetics centres

LONDON AREA

Kennedy Galton Centre
Northwick Park Hospital
Harrow
Middlesex

Clinical Genetics Unit
Institute of Child Health
30 Guilford Street
London WC1N 1EA

Paediatric Research Unit
Guy's Hospital
London SE1 9RT

Regional Genetics Service
St George's Hospital
London SW17 ORE

EAST ANGLIA

Genetics Counselling Service
Addenbrooke's Hospital
Cambridge CB2 2QQ

OXFORD

Department of Medical Genetics
Churchill Hospital
Headington
Oxford OX3 7LD

MERSEY

Regional Genetics Counselling Service
Countess of Chester Hospital
Chester CH2 2BA

Regional Genetic Counselling Service
Royal Liverpool Hospital
PO Box 147
Liverpool L69 3BX

NORTH

Department of Medical Genetics
St Mary's Hospital
Hathersage Road
Manchester M13 0JH

Department of Clinical Genetics
Royal Manchester Children's Hospital
Manchester M27 1HA

Department of Human Genetics
University of Newcastle
19 Claremont Place
Newcastle upon Tyne NE1 4LP

Department of Clinical Genetics
Ashley Wing
St James Hospital
Leeds LS2 7TF

MIDLANDS

West Midlands Regional Genetics
  Service
Birmingham Maternity Hospital
Edgbaston
Birmingham B15 2TH

Regional Genetics Services
East Birmingham Hospital
Bordesley Green East
Birmingham B9 5ST

Department of Clinical Genetics
Leicester Royal Infirmary
Leicester LE1 5WW

Centre for Human Genetics
17 Manchester Road
Sheffield S10 5DN

SOUTH

Regional Cytogenetics Service
Southmead Hospital
Bristol BS10 5NB

Clinical Genetics Department
Royal Hospital for Sick Children
St Michael's Hill
Bristol B52 5BJ

Regional Genetics Service
Bowmore House
Royal Devon and Exeter Hospital
(Wonford)
Barrack Road
Exeter EX2 5DW

Regional Genetics Service
Princess Anne Hospital
Coxford Road
Southampton SO9 4HA

WALES

Institute of Medical Genetics
University Hospital of Wales
Heath Park
Cardiff CF4 4XN

SCOTLAND

Human Genetics Unit
Western General Hospital
Crewe Road
Edinburgh EH4 2XU

Duncan Guthrie Institute of Medical
Genetics
Royal Hospital for Sick Children
Yorkhill
Glasgow G3 8SJ

Regional Genetics Service
Department of Pathology
Ninewells Hospital
Dundee DD1 9SY

Regional Genetics Service
Raigmore Hospital
Inverness IV2 3UJ

NORTHERN IRELAND

Department of Medical Genetics
Belfast City Hospital
Belfast BT9 7AB

Appendix C: Glossary

Acute Sudden onset of symptoms of disease.

Adenoma sebaceum Specific rash found in tuberous sclerosis.

Aetiology The origin, causation and development of disease.

Amblyopia Reduced vision due to squint.

Amniocentesis Removal of amniotic fluid from around the foetus through the abdominal and uterine walls.

Amniotic fluid Fluid surrounding foetus in the uterus.

Antibiotic Drugs used against bacterial infections.

Asymptomatic No obvious signs of a disease process.

Ataxia Loss of control of voluntary movement.

Atresia Occlusion of a normal channel in the body.

Atrial septal defects Opening between the two upper chambers of the heart.

Atrophy Wasting of any part of the body.

Audiometry Specialized test for hearing.

Autism Developmental disorder affecting communication and social skills.

Autonomic nervous system Part of nervous system having control of routine bodliy functions.

Autosomal Concerned with bodily cells.

Avascular necrosis Death of tissue due to lack of blood supply.

Biopsy Removal of a small part of an organ tissue for diagnostic purposes.

Bronchiectasis Lung disease following infection, often sustained in childhood.

Cataracts Clouding of the lens of the eye.

Centile charts Standardized growth charts (height, weight and head circumference) for children.

Choanal atresia Congenital blocking of one, or both, nostrils.

Chorionic villus sampling Antenatal test performed on minute parts of placental tissue.

Chromosome Units of inheritance of which there are normally 46 in humans.

Chronic Long-standing disease.

Chronological age Age from date of birth.

Cilia Tiny hair-like structures found in many hollow organs of the body.

Co-arctation Narrowing of the aorta.

Colomba Developmental gaps in various parts of the eye.

Conductive deafness Specialized type of deafness not involving the nerves of hearing.

Consanguinity Close family relationship.

Cornea Transparent covering of the front of the eye.

Dermatologist Medical practitioner specializing in diseases of the skin.

Developmental age Stage of childhood development – not necessarily the same as the chronological age.

Diabetes Disease of the pancreas resulting in a dangerously high blood sugar.

Dialysis Method of removing waste-products from the body in the event of kidney failure.

Dyslexia A specific reading difficulty.

ECG Electrocardiogram, measuring the electrical activity of the heart.

EEG Electroencephalogram, measuring the electrical activity of the brain.

Endocarditis Infection of the inner lining of the heart.

Enzyme Complex organic substance causing chemical reactions in the body.

Epicanthic fold Folds of skin from the upper eyelid over inner edge of the eye.

Epiphyseal plates Growing parts of the bone.

Eustachian tube Tiny tube leading from the middle ear to the back of the throat.

Fallot's tetralogy Special type of congenital heart disease.

Febrile convulsions Convulsions due to a high fever in children under the age of five years.

Fistula An abnormal connection between two organs of the body, or between an organ and the exterior.

Fontanelle Gaps in the bones of young babies' skulls, covered by fibrous tissue.

Gene The ultimate units of inheritance found on the chromosomes.

Glaucoma Raised pressure in the eyeball due to a fault in the drainage system.

Hernia A weakening of muscular tissue allowing organs to protude.

Horseshoe kidney Type of congenital developmental abnormality.

Hydramnios Excess amount of amniotic fluid.

Hydrocephalus Abnormal increase of cerebrospinal fluid in the brain.

Hydrotherapy Special type of physiotherapy undertaken in water.

Hyperactivity Extreme activity in childhood.

Hypertension High blood pressure.

Hypertonic Increased muscular tone.

Hypertrophy Excess growth of a particular tissue.

Hyperventilation Over-breathing.

Hypocalcaemia Low blood levels of calcium.

Hypoglycaemia Low blood sugar.

Hypospadias Abnormal opening of urethra on the penis.

Hypothyroidism Under-function of the thyroid gland.

Hypotonic Decreased muscular tone.

Hypsarrhythmia Particular type of convulsions.

Inguinal Pertaining to the groin region.

Intercostal muscles Muscles between the ribs.

Iris Coloured part of the eye.

Jaundice Yellow coloration of the skin in liver disease.

Kyphosis Bending of the spine in an anterior-posterior manner.

Lordosis Normal curve of spine in region of the lower back.

Mainstream schools Schools catering for majority of children.

Meconium ileus Blockage of the small intestine in the new-born.

Meiosis Type of cell division producing sex cells.

Melanin Substance causing skin pigmentation.

Metabolism Chemical processes necessary to maintain life and health.

Microcephaly A small under-developed brain.

Mitosis Type of cell division producing similar cells.

Mutations Changes producing new effects.

Myringotomy Surgical procedure to withdraw excess fluid from the middle ear.

Naevi Small pigmented areas in the skin ('moles').

Nasogastric feeding Feeding through a tube passed into the stomach via the nose.

Nystagmus Jerky sideways or vertical, involuntary movements of the eyes.

Ophthalmolgist Medical practitioner specializing in diseases of the eye.

Opthalmoscope Instrument used to examine structures at the back of the eye.

Parathyroid Endocrine gland situated at the back of the thyroid gland.

Parietal bones One of the bones making up the skull (situated at each side of the head).

Patent ductus Specialized type of congenital heart disease in which there is a duct between the aorta and the pulmonary artery.

Perthes disease Disease of the hip in childhood.

Phalanges Bones of the fingers.

Photophobia Dislike of light.

Plantar response Reflex action of the toes when the sole of the foot is stimulated.

Platelets Structures in the blood necessary for proper clotting.

Ptosis Partial paralysis of the eyelids.

Pyloric stenosis Abnormality at the lower end of the stomach.

Pyridoxine A vitamin of the B group.

Radius One of the bones of the forearm.

Reflexes Involuntary responses occuring when specific parts of the body are stimulated.

Respite care Short-term care by paid volunteers, for disabled children.

Retina Tissue at the back of the eye (necessary for vision).

Scoliosis Sideways bending of the spine.

Sensori-neural deafness Deafness due to problems with the nerves of hearing.

Sinusitis Infection of the para-nasal sinuses.

Situs invertus Organs on the opposite side of the body to normal.

Sporadic Condition occurring in isolated cases.

Sprengal shoulder One shoulder higher than the other.

Systemic Condition relating to whole bodily system or group of organs.

Talipes Defect in the ankle – esrstwhile known as 'club-foot'.

Testosterone Male sex hormone.

Thrombosis Clotting of blood.

Thyroid Endocrine gland situated in the front of the neck.

Thyroxine Hormone secreted by the throid gland.

Tics Involuntary movements of the face or body.

Trachea Wind-pipe – conducts air from the nose and mouth to the bronchi.

Tracheostomy An artificial opening made in the trachea.

Ultra-sound Diagnostic test using ultra-high frequency sound waves to produce an image.

Urethra Opening of the bladder to the exterior.

Venepuncture Collection of blood from a vein.

Ventricular septal defect Congenital abnormality in which the two lower chambers of the heart are connected.

Wilm's Tumour Specialized tumour of the kidney.

Index

This index should be used, in addition to the normal function, as part of the referencing structure of the book. For example, the distribution of 'deafness' or 'heart defect' amongst the various syndromes can be readily seen. Thus the identification of a specific syndrome, knowing only some features, can be more easily determined.